GLUTEN FREE BAKING

The Easy, Step-by-step Instructions and Delicious Recipes

(The Gluten-free Cookbook for Beginners – Super Easy Recipes)

Penny Knisely

Published by Sharon Lohan

Gluten Free Baking: The Easy, Step-by-step Instructions and Delicious Recipes (The Gluten-free Cookbook for Beginners – Super Easy Recipes)

ISBN 978-1-990334-13-9

Legal & Disclaimer

Table of contents

Part 1

Chapter 1- Enjoy Gluten free slow cooker recipes

If you are in love with winters then you must also want to have good food in winters as well. Such comfort foods will help you out in making your winter evenings delightful. It would be even better for you to have all your favorite recipes on your dining table just out of slow cooker. It means you just have to put all of your ingredients in slow cooker and you will get yummy cooked food out of it in a very short interval of time. In winter, when you do not want to work so much, your slow cooker will definitely help you out in making delicious recipes for you by investing not so much hardships.

Many of you would like to have gluten free slow cooker recipes with you so that you can enjoy your winters on full extent. The gluten free recipes have become so much popular and you will love them all while learning all of these in this book. After that, you will love to have a gluten free lifestyle in your lives.

I am sure that all of these recipes would be loved y you a lot and once you get few of them even after trying in your kitchen, you will definitely love to try all of them at your home. You will be thinking that it sounds pretty much good to have gluten free recipes as a part of your daily diet.

It is quite possible that you will be trying all of them for the first time as you were not aware of them as before.

If you think that you are now going to have every meal free of gluten then what has been remaining after to eat now? Your answer is, you are still able to eat plenty of amazing recipes and foods even if you say no to gluten. Do not worry of the things that you cannot eat gluten and you are left with nothing. You can still have so much delicious dishes to eat which are having no gluten.

I have written this book to get you introduced with all those recipes which are free of gluten, are cooked in slow cooker, are very much easy to be followed and can provide good taste to your taste buds.

These recipes are super easy that you can have them done in a very short span of time with little investment of hard work. Especially in winters, when you are not willing to work more, these recipes would work for you very easily.

Your slow cooker will become your best friend which cooks delicious foods for you free of gluten. I am not fully aware of the extent of busyness you have but I am sure that even if you are busy in doing other things, you will definitely have something that can cook foods for you in no time. Yes, it is your slow cooker. I am going to share very simple and easy recipes which you can try at your home just by putting all of the ingredients I slow cooker.

All you need is slow cooker and the ingredients which I am going to elaborate in each recipe step by step. Switch on the stove by putting all the ingredients in it

3

and let the cocker do its job. You will come out with delicious and easy dishes which will suit your taste buds and help you out in eating all the healthy recipes which are gluten free.

So, here I go telling you all the delicious recipes in my book which you will love definitely and I hope you will try them as well.

Chapter 2- 27 Super Gluten Free slow cooker recipes (Chicken)

Buffalo Chicken with Egg plant

- Chicken boneless 1 kg
- Chili sauce 2 tablespoon
- Oil 1 tablespoon
- Soy sauce 1 teaspoon

Method:

- Mix all ingredients.
- Place in slow cooker.
- Cook till hot.

☐ **Nutritional facts:** Water, mineral and carbohydrates content is high

☐ **Calories:** 40 calories/ 100 g

Pepperoni Chicken

Ingredients:
- Chicken boneless half kg
- Black pepper 1 teaspoon
- Pizza sauce 2 tablespoon
- Oil 1 tablespoon

Method:
- Combine all ingredients.
- Cook in slow cooker till chicken becomes soft.
- Enjoy.

☐ **Nutritional facts:** Animal fat, low in Carbohydrates, minerals
☐ **Calories:** 60 calories/ 100 g

Thai chicken with vegetable spring onion

Ingredients:
- Chicken boiled half kg
- Mixed vegetables 1 cup
- Spring onion boiled 1 packet
- Thai spices 2 tablespoon

Method:
- Cook all ingredients in slow cooker except spring onion.
- Serve by placing the dish over spring onion.

☐ **Nutritional facts:** Low in carbohydrates and high in vitaminss, just suitable for a gluten free diet.
☐ **Calories:** 35 calories/ 100 g

Apricot chicken

- Chicken boneless 1 kg
- Canned apricots with syrup 1 cup
- Barbeque sauce 2 tablespoon
- Thyme a pinch

Method:

- Mix all ingredients.
- Put in slow cooker and cook till hot.
- Serve.

☐ **Nutritional facts:** Low in Carbohydrates a lot of mineral content.

☐ **Calories:** 40 calories/ 100 g

Creamy Crock-Pot Chicken with

Ingredients:
- Chicken half kg
- Cream whipped 100 grams
- Mayonnaise 100 grams
- Milk half cup
- Black pepper 2 teaspoon

Method:
- Mix chicken with all ingredients.
- Put in slow cooker till hot.
- Enjoy.

☐ **Nutritional facts:** Low in carbohydrates and high in vitaminss, just suitable for a gluten free diet.
☐ **Calories:** 70 calories/ 100 g

Slow Cooker Creamy Chicken

Ingredients:
- Chicken boneless 1 kg
- Whipped cream half cup
- Tomato puree half cup
- Barbeque sauce 4 tablespoon

Method:
- Marinate chicken with all the sauces and cream.
- Leave for half an hour.
- Cook in slow cooker till chicken becomes soft.
- Serve.

☐ **Nutritional facts:**Low in Carbohydrates, the rich use of tomato can add a lot of mineral content.

☐ **Calories:** 45 calories/ 100 g

Slow-Pot Chicken with mushrooms

Ingredients:
- Chicken boneless 500 grams
- Thyme a pinch
- Worchester sauce 3 tablespoon
- Onion 2 chopped

Method:
- Make onions fry in slow cooker till brown.
- Add rest of ingredients.
- Cook till chicken becomes tender.

☐ **Nutritional facts:** Full of vitamins with moderate content of carbohydrates

☐ **Calories:** 60 calories/ 100 g

Gluten-Free Crock-Pot

Ingredients:

- Chicken stock half cup
- Chicken boneless half kg
- Black pepper and salt as required
- Spring onion chopped 1 cup
- Barbeque sauce 4 tablespoon
- Oil 2 tablespoon
- Jalapeno chopped 2

Method:

- Take chicken stock in cooker till boiled.
- Add rest of the ingredients as well.
- Cook in slow cooker till chicken becomes tender.

☐ **Nutritional facts:** Abundance of vitamins. Thevegetables can be a healthy addition.
☐ **Calories:** 35 calories/ 100 g

Chicken barbeque hearts

Ingredients:
- Chicken mince half kg
- Barbeque sauce 4 tablespoon
- Oil 2 tablespoon
- Corn flour 2 tablespoon

Method:
- Mix all ingrains in chicken mince except oil.
- Make heart shaped nuggets.
- Cook in slow cooker till hot.

☐ **Nutritional facts:** Excessive carbohydrates and fiber content, is especially useful for all the gluten free plans.
☐ **Calories:** 45 calories/ 100 g

Chicken Fajitas

Ingredients:
- Chicken boneless half kg
- Fajita sauce 4 tablespoon
- Oil 2 tablespoon

Method:
- Combine all ingredients.
- Cook till hot.
- Enjoy.

☐ **Nutritional facts:** High mineral content and rich in animal fat, low in Carbohydrates
☐ **Calories:** 20 calories/ 100 g

Oriental slow cookerChicken

Ingredients:

- Chicken 1 kg
- Red pepper flakes 2 teaspoon
- Onion chopped 1 cup
- Oil 2 tablespoon
- Salt and vinegar 2 teaspoon each

Method:

- Marinate chicken with all the ingredients.
- Put it along with oil in slow cooker.
- Cook till hot.
- Serve.

☐ **Nutritional facts:** Vitamins and fiber content is nil, low in carbohydrates and high in minerals, just suitable for a gluten free diet.

☐ **Calories:** 40 calories/ 100 g

Spicy chicken

Ingredients:
- Chicken half kg boneless
- Red pepper flakes 2 teaspoon
- Hot sauce 1 tablespoon
- Corn flour 1 tablespoon
- Oil 3 tablespoon

Method:
- Mix all ingredients in cooker.
- Cook till hot.
- **Nutritional facts:** Rich in fat, low in Carbohydrates, the rich use of sauces can add a lot of mineral content.
- **Calories:** 30 calories/ 100 g

Peach chicken

Ingredients:
- Peach with syrup 1 tin
- Chicken 1 kg
- Black pepper 1 teaspoon
- Soy sauce 2 teaspoon
- Oil 2 tablespoon

Method:
- Mix all ingredients.
- Cook in slow cooker.
- Serve.

☐ **Nutritional facts:** Vitamins, fat and carbohydrates
☐ **Calories:** 50 calories/ 100 g

Cashew chicken

Ingredients:
- Cashew nuts roasted 1 cup
- Chicken half kg
- Salt 1 teaspoon
- Soy sauce 2 teaspoon
- Oil 4 tablespoon

Method:
- Combine all ingredients in cooker.
- Cook till chicken becomes tender.

☐ **Nutritional facts:** Vitamins, fat and carbohydrates
☐ **Calories:** 74 calories/ 100 g

Sweet and Spicy Chicken

Ingredients:

- Hot sauce 1 teaspoon
- Chili sauce 2 tablespoon
- Chicken half kg
- Black pepper 1 teaspoon
- Olive oil 2 tablespoon

Method:

- Mix all ingredients.
- Marinate for half an hour.
- Cook till hot.

☐ **Nutritional facts:** Water, mineral and carbohydrate content is high

☐ **Calories:** 70 calories/ 100 g

Chicken tikka special

Ingredients:
- Tikka spices 4 tablespoon
- Barbeque sauce 2 teaspoon
- Soy sauce 1 tablespoon
- Chicken 1 kg
- Garlic paste 2 teaspoon

Method:
- Mix all ingredients and marinate chicken for 2 hours.
- Cook till chicken becomes soft.
- Serve.

☐ **Nutritional facts:** Water, mineral and carbohydrate content is high

☐ **Calories:** 87 calories/ 100 g

Chicken Teriyaki

Ingredients:
- Teriyaki sauce 2 tablespoon
- Chicken boneless 1 kg
- Vinegar 1 teaspoon

Method:
- Mix all ingredients with chicken.
- Add oil to cooker, add chicken in to it.
- Cook till hot.

☐ **Nutritional facts:** Vitamins, fat and carbohydrates
☐ **Calories:** 70 calories/ 100 g

Chicken with cauliflower

Ingredients:
- Cauliflower roasted 1 cup
- Oil 2 teaspoon
- Chicken half kg
- Ginger garlic paste 2 teaspoon
- Chopped spring onion half cup

Method:
- Stir fry ginger garlic paste and onions till brown.
- Add rest of ingredients.
- Cook till chicken gets completely cooked.

☐ **Nutritional facts:** Water, mineral and carbohydrate content is high

☐ **Calories:** 98 calories/ 100 g

Chicken lettuce

Ingredients:
- Lettuce 1 cup chopped
- Chicken 1 kg boiled
- Black pepper 1 teaspoon
- Tomatoes chopped 2
- Oil 2 tablespoon

Method:
- Stir fry lettuce in oil.
- Add chicken till golden.
- Add rest of ingredients.
- Cook in slow cooker till hot.

☐ **Nutritional facts:** Water, mineral and carbohydrate content is high
☐ **Calories:** 65 calories/ 100 g

Swiss chicken steaks

Ingredients:
- Chicken steaks half kg
- Barbeque sauce 3 tablespoon
- Oil 2 tablespoon
- Oregano 1 teaspoon
- Black pepper 1 teaspoon

Method:
- Marinate chicken with all ingredients.
- Add oil to cooker.
- Add chicken and cook till hot.

☐ **Nutritional facts:** Vitamins, fat and carbohydrates
☐ **Calories:** 76 calories/ 100 g

Chicken meatballs with BBQ sauce

Ingredients:
- Chicken mince half kg
- Red pepper 1 teaspoon
- Salt as required
- Barbeque sauce 2 tablespoon
- Oil to fry

Method:
- Combine all ingredients with chicken mince.
- Make small balls.
- Fry in cooker with oil until soft.

☐ **Nutritional facts:** Water, mineral and carbohydrate content is high
☐ **Calories:** 75 calories/ 100 g

Chicken slow cooker roast

Ingredients:
- Chicken full 1
- Barbeque sauce 2 tablespoon
- Oil 2 tablespoon
- Yogurt half cup
- Cream 2 tablespoon

Method:
- Combine all ingredients.
- Marinate chicken.
- Cook in slow cooker till hot.

☐ **Nutritional facts:** Water, mineral and carbohydrate content is high

☐ **Calories:** 63 calories/ 100 g

Chicken with peanut butter

Ingredients:

- Peanut butter half cup
- Chicken boneless half kg
- Salt 1 teaspoon
- Black pepper 2 teaspoon

Method:

- Mix all ingredients in slow cooker.
- Switch on the stove and cook till hot.

☐ **Nutritional facts:** Vitamins and carbohydrates
☐ **Calories:** 30 calories/ 100 g

Spicy chicken mince

Ingredients:
- Spring onion boiled 1 packet
- Chicken mince 1 kg
- Hot sauce 2 tablespoon

Method:
- Combine all ingredients except spring onion.
- Make meatballs and cook in cooker.
- Put balls with sauce over spring onion.
- Serve.

☐ **Nutritional facts:** Water, mineral and carbohydrate content is high

☐ **Calories:** 87 calories/ 100 g

Chicken roast with green chilies

Ingredients:
- Chicken half kg
- Green chilies 4 chopped
- Oil 3 tablespoon
- Barbeque sauce 2 tablespoon

Method:
- Add oil to cooker and rest of ingredients.
- Cook till hot.
- Add chilies at end.
- Serve.

☐ **Nutritional facts:** Water, mineral and carbohydrate content is high
☐ **Calories:** 86 calories/ 100 g

Soy chicken roast

Ingredients:
- Soy sauce 2 tablespoon
- Chicken 1 kg
- Black and red pepper flakes
- Oil 2 tablespoon
- Oregano a pinch

Method:
- Marinate chicken with all ingredients except oil.
- Put oil in cooker.
- Cook slowly till hot.

☐ **Nutritional facts:** Water, mineral and carbohydrate content is high
☐ **Calories:** 23 calories/ 100 g

Habanero Chili Chicken:

- Red chili powder 1 teaspoon
- Chicken 800 grams
- Habanero sauce 2 teaspoon
- Oil 2 tablespoon
- Mustard paste 2 teaspoon

Method:

- Combine all spices and sauces with chicken.
- Marinate for an hour.
- Add oil in cooker and add chicken.
- Cook till hot.

☐ **Nutritional facts:** Water, mineral and carbohydrate content is high

☐ **Calories:** 70 calories/ 100 g

Chapter 3- 41Super Gluten Free slow cooker recipes (Goat and Beef)

Slow cooked spicy beef

Ingredients:
- Beef boneless half kg
- Hot and chili sauce 2 tablespoon each
- Red chili flakes 2 teaspoon
- Salt as required

Method:
- Combine all ingredients with beef.
- Leave for two hours.
- Put in slow cooker.
- Cook till tender.

☐ **Nutritional facts:** Vitamins, fat and carbohydrates
☐ **Calories:** 71 calories/ 100 g

Beef black pepper mince

Ingredients:
- Beef mince 1 kg
- Black and white pepper 1 teaspoon each
- Mustard powder 2 tablespoon
- Barbeque sauce half cup

Method:
- Combine all ingredients except barbeque sauce.
- Make balls and cook slowly.
- Add barbeque sauce at end.

☐ **Nutritional facts:** Water, mineral and carbohydrate content is high

☐ **Calories:** 85 calories/ 100 g

Slow cooked beef roast

- Beef half kg
- Barbeque and soy sauce 2 tablespoon each
- Oil 2 tablespoon
- Vinegar 2 tablespoon

Method:

- Mix all ingredients in cooker.
- Cook till hot in slow cooker.

☐ **Nutritional facts:** Water, mineral and carbohydrate content is high

☐ **Calories:** 49 calories/ 100 g

Worchester beef meatballs

- Beef 1 kg minced
- Worchester sauce 4 tablespoon

Method:

- Combine both ingredients.
- Make small balls.
- Cook slowly in cooker.
- **Nutritional facts:** Water, mineral and carbohydrate content is high
- **Calories:** 84 calories/ 100 g

Spicy beef casserole

- Beef half kg
- Hot sauce 2 tablespoon
- Mayonnaise 1 cup
- Salt as required

Method:

- Combine all ingredients.
- Cook in slow cooker till hot.

☐ **Nutritional facts:** Minerals, carbohydrates and water content is high

☐ **Calories:**65 calories/ 100 g

Orange beef

- Beef boneless half kg
- Orange juice 1 cup
- Orange food color 1 teaspoon
- All spices 2 teaspoon

Method:

Combine all ingredients.

Cook slowly till hot.

☐ **Nutritional facts:** Vitamins, fats.

☐ **Calories:** 90 calories/ 100 g

Slow cooker beef curry

- Beef 1 kg
- Corn flour 2 teaspoon
- Ketchup 4 tablespoon
- Red pepper 1 teaspoon

Method:

- Combine all ingredients.
- Cook in slow cooker till hot.
- Enjoy.

☐ **Nutritional facts:** Water, mineral and carbohydrate content is high

☐ **Calories:** 77 calories/ 100 g

Beef with apricots

- Apricots canned 1 cup
- Beef boiled boneless half kg
- Black pepper 2 teaspoon

Method:

- Add all ingredients in slow cooker.
- Cook till hot.

☐ **Nutritional facts:** Minerals, carbohydrates and water content is high

☐ **Calories:**87 calories/ 100 g

Beef spicy curry

- Beef boneless 1 kg
- Oil 2 tablespoon
- Beef stock half cup
- Barbeque sauce 2 tablespoon

Method:

- Combine all ingredients.
- Cook in slow cooker.

☐ **Nutritional facts:** Minerals, carbohydrates and water content is high

☐ **Calories:**76 calories/ 100 g

Italian beef

- Italian herbs 2 tablespoon
- Slat as required
- Beef boneless half kg

Method:
- Combine all ingredients in slow cooker.
- Cook till beef becomes tender.

☐ **Nutritional facts:** Water, mineral and carbohydrate content is high

☐ **Calories:** 95 calories/ 100 g

Fajita beef

- Beef boneless and boiled 1 kg
- Fajita sauce 2 tablespoon
- Oil 2 tablespoon

Method:
- Combine all ingredients.
- Cook in slow cooker till completely cooked.

☐ **Nutritional facts:** Vitamins, fat and carbohydrates
☐ **Calories:** 60 calories/ 100 g

Slow cooker beef mince

- Beef mince half kg
- Black and white pepper 2 teaspoon
- Onion chopped 1 medium

Method:

- Add onion in slow cooker.
- Followed by all other ingredients.
- Cook slowly till hot.

☐ **Nutritional facts:** Minerals, carbohydrates and water content is high

☐ **Calories:**65 calories/ 100 g

Corn beef

- Sweet corn 1 cup
- Beef boiled 400 grams
- Soy sauce 3 tablespoon

Method:

- Combine all ingredients in slow cooker.
- Cook till hot.

☐ **Nutritional facts:** Water, mineral and carbohydrate content is high

☐ **Calories:** 63 calories/ 100 g

Slow cooked beef with vegetables

- Mixed vegetables 1 cup roasted
- Beef mince 1 cup boiled
- Barbeque and Worcestershire sauce 2 tablespoon

Method:

- Add all ingredients in slow cooker.
- Cook till tender.

☐ **Nutritional facts:** Vitamins, fat and carbohydrates
☐ **Calories:** 98 calories/ 100 g

Easy slow cooked beef

- Beef half kg boneless
- Vinegar 2 tablespoon
- Soy sauce and pepper 2 teaspoon
- Spring onion chopped 1 cup

Method:

- Mix all ingredients in cooker.
- Cook till hot.

☐ **Nutritional facts:** Water, mineral and carbohydrate content is high

☐ **Calories:** 67 calories/ 100 g

Taco beef

- Beef 1 kg
- Taco sauce 2 tablespoon
- Soy sauce 3 tablespoon
- Ginger garlic paste 2 tablespoon

Method:

- Mix ginger garlic paste with beef.
- Marinate for 2 hours.
- Add rest of ingredients.
- Cook slowly till soft.

☐ **Nutritional facts:** Minerals, carbohydrates and water content is high

☐ **Calories:**87 calories/ 100 g

Beef with roasted green beans

- Beef 1 kg boiled boneless
- Green beans roasted 1 cup
- Barbeque sauce 2 tablespoon

Method:

- Cook all ingredients in slow cooker till hot.
- Enjoy.

☐ **Nutritional facts:** Vitamins, fat and carbohydrates
☐ **Calories:** 40 calories/ 100 g

Asian slow cooked beef

- Beef 1 kg
- All spices 2 tablespoon
- Red pepper 2 teaspoon
- Tomato paste 4 tablespoon

Method:

- Combine all ingredients in slow cooker.
- Cook till hot.

☐ **Nutritional facts:** Minerals, carbohydrates and water content is high

☐ **Calories:**40 calories/ 100 g

Crispy beef Pattie

Ingredients:
- Boneless beef boiled 1 cup
- Potato boiled 1 cup
- Soy sauce and pepper 1 teaspoon
- Mustard sauce 2 tablespoon

Method:
- Combine all ingredients and make egg like in shape.
- Cook in slow cooker.
- Enjoy.

☐ **Nutritional facts:** Vitamins, fat and carbohydrates
☐ **Calories:** 65 calories/ 100 g

Potato and corn beef

Ingredients:
- Potato boiled 2
- Canned corns half can
- Beef 500 grams boneless
- Oil 3 tablespoon
- Barbeque sauce 2 tablespoon

Method:
- Take all ingredients in cooker.
- Stir fry first.
- Then add water and cook till meat becomes tender.
- Enjoy.

☐ **Nutritional facts:** Water, mineral and carbohydrate content is high

☐ **Calories:** 63 calories/ 100 g

Stuffed meat balls

Ingredients:
- Beef mince 1 cup
- Jalapeno and onion chopped 2
- Oregano a pinch
- Cheese 200 grams

Method:
- Mix all ingredients except cheese and make tiny balls.
- Stuff cheese inside and cover it again.
- Cook slowly.

☐ **Nutritional facts:** Minerals, carbohydrates and water content is high

☐ **Calories:**98 calories/ 100 g

Beef with red beans

Ingredients:
- Red beans boiled 1 cup
- Beef boneless 500 grams
- Barbeque sauce 2 tablespoon

Method:
- Boil all the ingredients together in slow cooker.
- Till water dries and beef becomes soft.
- Enjoy.

☐ **Nutritional facts:** Water, mineral and carbohydrate content is high

☐ **Calories:** 91 calories/ 100 g

Ginger stir-fried beef

Ingredients:
- Beef steaks 2 chopped
- Ginger paste 2 tablespoon
- Oil 2 tablespoon
- Soy sauce 1 teaspoon

Method:

Combine all ingredients in cooker.

Cook till hot.

☐ **Nutritional facts:** Vitamins, fat and carbohydrates

☐ **Calories:** 30 calories/ 100 g

Beef steaks

Ingredients:
- Beef steaks smoked 2
- Bread crumbs to coat
- Egg 1
- Soy sauce and barbeque sauce 2 tablespoon each
- Salt as required

Method:
- Combine steaks chopped with sauces and salt.
- Coat them with egg then with bread crumbs.
- Cook till hot.

☐ **Nutritional facts:** Water, mineral and carbohydrate content is high

☐ **Calories:** 10 calories/ 100 g

Tasty beef casserole with cheese

Ingredients:
- Potato and capsicum 2 each
- Oil 2 tablespoon
- Cheese 1 cup
- Barbeque sauce 3 tablespoon

Method:
- Combine all ingredients in pan except cheese.
- Dish it out.
- Add cheese from top.

☐ **Nutritional facts:** Minerals, carbohydrates and water content is high

☐ **Calories:**98 calories/ 100 g

Beef balls

- Oregano 1 teaspoon
- Flour 1 cup
- Oil 2 teaspoon
- White pepper half teaspoon
- Salt as required
- Eggs 2 beaten
- Beef boiled 1 cup

Method:
- Combine all ingredients in a bowl.
- Make balls shaped and cook slowly.
- Serve.

☐ **Nutritional facts:** Minerals, carbohydrates and water content is high
☐ **Calories:**76 calories/ 100 g

- Beef quiche for Paleo diet
- Beef boiled half cup
- Cottage cheese 1 cup

- Olive oil half teaspoon
- White pepper half teaspoon

Method:
- Add spinach with oil in cooker.
- Add cheese and pepper.
- Cook till hot.

☐ **Nutritional facts:** Vitamins, fat and carbohydrates
☐ **Calories:** 97 calories/ 100 g

Italian beef frittata

- Tomatoes 1 chopped
- Olive oil half teaspoon
- Eggs 3
- Salt and pepper as required
- Shredded beef 1 cup

Method:

- Beat all ingredients with eggs.
- Add olive oil.
- Cook slowly till hot.

☐ **Nutritional facts:** Minerals, carbohydrates and water content is high

☐ **Calories:**87 calories/ 100 g

Beef potato curry

Ingredients:
- Boneless beef half kg
- Potato 2
- Ginger paste 2 tablespoon
- Barbeque sauce 2 tablespoon
- Salt to taste
- Oil 2 tablespoon

Method:
- Add all ingredients in slow cooker.
- Cook till becomes soft.

☐ **Nutritional facts:** Water, mineral and carbohydrate content is high

☐ **Calories:** 96 calories/ 100 g

Sweet potato hash browns with beef

- Sweet potatoes boiled 2
- Beef boiled shredded half cup
- Mayonnaise half cup

Method:

- Add potatoes to oil in cooker.
- Cook till brown.
- Add rest of ingredients.
- Enjoy.

☐ **Nutritional facts:** Water, mineral and carbohydrate content is high

☐ **Calories:** 87 calories/ 100 g

Russian omelet

- Capsicum 1 chopped
- Apple 1 chopped
- Peas boiled half cup
- Eggs 2 beaten
- Cream 2 teaspoon
- Beef shredded half cup

Method:

- Add all ingredients to cooker.
- Cook slowly till cooked well.

☐ **Nutritional facts:** Vitamins, fat and carbohydrates
☐ **Calories:** 40 calories/ 100 g

Spring onion beef

Ingredients:
- Beef shredded 1 cup
- Spring onions chopped 1 cup
- Cheese 100 grams

Method:
- Combine all ingredients except cheese.
- Add oil in pan and cook till hot.
- Add cheese at end till it melts.

☐ **Nutritional facts:** Water, mineral and carbohydrate content is high

☐ **Calories:** 40 calories/ 100 g

Veggie soup with beef

- Mixed vegetables 1 cup
- Chicken stock 1 cup
- Corn flour 2 tablespoon
- Beef half cup shredded

Method:

- Add all ingredients in slow cooker.
- Cook till hot.
- Add corn flour.
- Cook till thickens.

☐ **Nutritional facts:** Water, mineral and carbohydrate content is high

☐ **Calories:** 71 calories/ 100 g

Classic Greek beef salad

- Cabbage 1 cup
- Onion half cup
- Vinegar 4 tablespoon
- Red pepper half teaspoon
- Olives half cup
- Tomatoes half cup

Method:

- Cook beef in slow cooker.
- Mix all ingredients followed by red pepper.
- **Nutritional facts:** Minerals, carbohydrates and water content is high
    - **Calories:**99 calories/ 100 g

Beef mayonnaise casserole

Ingredients:
- Mayonnaise 1 cup
- Beef boiled and shredded 1 cup
- Pepper and salt as required
- Soy sauce 2 tablespoon

Method:
- Add beef, pepper and salt in slow cooker with oil.
- Cook till soft.
- Add mayonnaise at end.
- Mix.

☐ **Nutritional facts:** Water, mineral and carbohydrate content is high

☐ **Calories:** 98 calories/ 100 g

Tasty beef casserole with cheese

Ingredients:

- Potato and capsicum 2 each
- Oil 2 tablespoon
- Cheese 1 cup
- Barbeque sauce 3 tablespoon

Method:

- Combine all ingredients in slow cooker except cheese.
- Dish it out.
- Add cheese from top.

☐ **Nutritional facts:** Vitamins, fat and carbohydrates
☐ **Calories:** 77 calories/ 100 g

Vegie beef Shashlik

- Mixed vegetables 1 cup
- Eggs 2
- Beef 1 cup shredded
- Oil 2 tablespoon
- Salt and white pepper as requires

Method:

- Beat eggs in bowl; fry the mixed vegetables in oil.
- Add rest of ingredients.
- Cook slowly until hot.

☐ **Nutritional facts:** Minerals, carbohydrates and water content is high

☐ **Calories:**99 calories/ 100 g

Beef rice

- Beef boiled 1 cup
- Rice boiled 1 cup
- Salt to taste
- Water one cup

Method:
- Half boil the rice.
- Add Beef to water till boil.
- Add half boiled rice along with vinegar and salt in to it.
- Cook in slow cooker till hot.

☐ **Nutritional facts:** Water, mineral and carbohydrate content is high
☐ **Calories:** 98 calories/ 100 g

Zucchini beef salad

- Beef half cup boiled
- Mixed vegetables one cup
- Cream half cup
- Cucumber 2 sliced

Method:

- Combine all ingredients.
- Cook beef in slow cooker.
- Serve refrigerated.

☐ **Nutritional facts:** Minerals, carbohydrates and water content is high

☐ **Calories:**67 calories/ 100 g

Savory beef salad

- Beef boiled 200 grams
- Cream whipped one cup
- Mayonnaise half cup
- White pepper half teaspoon
- Mixed vegetables 1 cup

Method:

- Take a bowl and combine all the ingredients.
- Cook beef in slow cooker.
- Mix them all.

☐ **Nutritional facts:** Vitamins, fat and carbohydrates
☐ **Calories:** 75 calories/ 100 g

Spinach rice with peer

Ingredients:
- Rice boiled 2 cups
- Spinach boiled half cup
- Chili sauce and salt as required

Method:
- Combine all ingredients except rice in pan.
- Cook in slow cooker till soft.
- Add rice at end.

☐ **Nutritional facts:** Water, mineral and carbohydrate content is high

☐ **Calories:** 47 calories/ 100 g

Chapter 4-22Super Gluten Free slow cooker recipes (Lamb)

Creamy lamb soup

Ingredients:

- Corn flour 2 tablespoon
- Ketchup 2 tablespoon
- Lamb boiled and roasted 1 cup
- Onion 1 medium chopped
- Vinegar 1 teaspoon

Method:

- Add water in slow cooker.
- Add rest of ingredients.
- Cook till hot.

☐ **Nutritional facts:** Vitamins, fat and carbohydrates
☐ **Calories:** 66 calories/ 100 g

Ginger garlic lamb spring onion

Ingredients:

- Spring onion 1 packet
- Barbeque sauce 2 teaspoon
- Chili sauce 1 tablespoon
- Ginger garlic paste 3 tablespoon
- Lamb boiled 1 cup

Method:

- Boil spring onion in water.
- Add all ingredients in slow cooker.
- Cook till hot.

☐ **Nutritional facts:** Minerals, carbohydrates and water content is high
☐ **Calories:**88 calories/ 100 g

Creamy slow cooked lamb

Ingredients:

- Fresh cream half cup
- Lamb mince 1 cup boiled
- Mayonnaise half cup

Method:

- Combine all the ingredients carefully in slow cooker.
- Cook till hot.

☐ **Nutritional facts:** Water, mineral and carbohydrate content is high
☐ **Calories:** 65 calories/ 100 g

Oregano lamb delight

Ingredients:

- Oregano 2 tablespoon
- Soy and chili sauce 2 teaspoon each
- White pepper to taste
- Boneless lamb meat 1 cup boiled

Method:

- Mix all the ingredients in slow cooker.
- Cook till hot.

☐ **Nutritional facts:** Vitamins, fat and carbohydrates
☐ **Calories:** 89 calories/ 100 g

Garlic slow cooked lamb with green chili

- Chicken half kg
- Garlic paste 3 tablespoon
- Salt as required
- Green chili chopped 4

Method:

- Mix all ingredients.
- Slow cook till hot.

☐ **Nutritional facts:** Minerals, carbohydrates and water content is high

☐ **Calories:**90 calories/ 100 g

Spring onion lamb chops

- Lamb chops 4
- Vinegar and soy sauce 2 teaspoon each
- All spices 2 teaspoon
- Salt to taste

Method:

- Marinate chops with all ingredients for an hour.
- Add onion with all other ingredients in slow cooker.
- Cook till hot.

☐ **Nutritional facts:** Minerals, carbohydrates and water content is high

☐ **Calories:**85 calories/ 100 g

Lamb burgundy

- Lamb boiled half kg
- Barbeque and soy sauce 2 tablespoon
- Oil to fry
- Bread crumbs to coat

Method:

- Marinate lamb with sauces.
- Coat it with bread crumbs.
- Cook in slow cooker till hot.

☐ **Nutritional facts:** Vitamins, fat and carbohydrates
☐ **Calories:** 65 calories/ 100 g

Slow cooked lamb with mushrooms

Ingredients:

- Mushrooms 1 can
- Capsicum 1 medium
- Barbeque sauce 2 tablespoon
- Salt as required
- Lamb boneless 1 kg

Method:

- Mix all ingredients in bowl.
- Cook in slow cooker till hot.

☐ **Nutritional facts:** Water, mineral and carbohydrate content is high
☐ **Calories:** 70 calories/ 100 g

Lamb stuffed mushrooms

- Lamb boiled 400 grams
- Mushrooms 200 grams
- Oil 2 teaspoon
- Barbeque sauce 2 tablespoon

Method:

- Marinate lamb with barbeque sauce.
- Add all ingredients in slow cooker.
- Cook till hot.

☐ **Nutritional facts:** Water, mineral and carbohydrate content is high

☐ **Calories:** 43 calories/ 100 g

Lamb Avocado

- Lamb mince boiled half kg
- Avocado half cup
- Black pepper and salt 1 teaspoon
- Oil 2 tablespoon

Method:

- Mix all ingredients slow cooker.
- Cook till hot.
- Enjoy.

☐ **Nutritional facts:** Water, mineral and carbohydrate content is high
☐ **Calories:** 40 calories/ 100 g

Creamy lamb mushroom curry

Ingredients:

- Fresh cream 1 cup
- Mayonnaise 1 cup
- Mushrooms half can
- Salt as required
- Lamb 1 cup boiled

Method:

- Combine all the ingredients with each other.
- Cook in slow cooker.
- Enjoy.

☐ **Nutritional facts:** Vitamins, fat and carbohydrates
☐ **Calories:** 99 calories/ 100 g

Stuffed lamb in capsicum

Ingredients:

- Capsicum 2 seedless
- Mayonnaise 2 tablespoon
- Boiled rice 1 cup
- Black pepper 1 teaspoon
- Lamb shredded 1 cup

Method:

- Mix all ingredients except capsicum.
- Fill the material inside capsicum.
- Cook in slow cooker till hot.

☐ **Nutritional facts:** Minerals, carbohydrates and water content is high
☐ **Calories:**88 calories/ 100 g

Lamb spice

- Oil 2 tablespoon
- Lamb boneless half kg
- All spices 1 teaspoon
- Ginger paste 1 teaspoon

Method:

- Add oil, ginger paste and chicken till it becomes softened.
- Add all spices and salt.
- Cook in slow cooker till hot.

☐ **Nutritional facts:** Minerals, carbohydrates and water content is high

☐ **Calories:**55 calories/ 100 g

Poached lamb with Pears

- Pears canned 100 grams
- Sugar syrup half cup
- Coco powder quarter cup
- Honey two tablespoon
- Boiled lamb 1 cup shredded

Method:

- Combine all ingredients together.
- Cook in slow cooker.

☐ **Nutritional facts:** Vitamins, fat and carbohydrates
☐ **Calories:** 86 calories/ 100 g

Lamb rice

- Boiled rice 1 cup
- Shredded Lamb 1 cup
- Salt and pepper to taste
- Oil 1 tablespoon

Method:

- Add oil, lamb, salt and pepper to slow cooker.
- Add rice at end.
- Cook till hot.

☐ **Nutritional facts:** Water, mineral and carbohydrate content is high

☐ **Calories:** 50 calories/ 100 g

Creamy Lamb salsa

Ingredients:
- Lamb boiled 1 kg
- Cream 100 gram
- Mayonnaise 50 gram
- Honey 2 tablespoon
- Salt to taste

Method:
- Mix all the ingredients in slow cooker.
- Cook till hot.

☐ **Nutritional facts:** Vitamins, fat and carbohydrates
☐ **Calories:** 50 calories/ 100 g

Spreader egg with lamb stuffed

Ingredients:
- Egg boiled 2
- Shredded lamb 1 cup
- White pepper and salt as required
- Mayonnaise 1 cup

Method:
- Mix all ingredients in a bowl except eggs.
- Fill the material in eggs.
- Cook in slow cooker till hot.

☐ **Nutritional facts:** Vitamins, fat and carbohydrates
☐ **Calories:** 95 calories/ 100 g

Crispy Lamb with chili

Ingredients:
- Lamb half kg
- Corn flour 2 tablespoon
- Oil to fry
- Soy sauce 1 teaspoon

Method:
- Coat Lamb with soy sauce, salt and corn floor.
- Cook in slow cooker till tender.

☐ **Nutritional facts:** Water, mineral and carbohydrate content is high

☐ **Calories:** 30 calories/ 100 g

Butter lamb

Ingredients:
- Butter 100 grams
- Lamb boiled 500 grams
- Black pepper and salt as required

Method:
- Add lamb, butter and spices in slow cooker.
- Cook till become consistent.

☐ **Nutritional facts:** Water, mineral and carbohydrate content is high

☐ **Calories:** 54 calories/ 100 g

Lamb fried rice

Ingredients:
- Rice 1 cup boiled
- Lamb 1 cup boiled
- All spiced 1 tablespoon
- Vinegar as required

Method:
- Combine all ingredients except rice.
- Add rice when hot.
- Mix them well.
- Cook in slow cooker till hot.

☐ **Nutritional facts:** Vitamins, fat and carbohydrates
☐ **Calories:** 20 calories/ 100 g

Lamb steaks with cheese

Ingredients:
- Cheddar cheese 1 cup
- Lamb steaks 4 smoked
- Chili and soy sauce 2 table spoon each
- Barbeque sauce 1 tablespoon

Method:
- Combine all ingredients in slow cooker.
- Cook till hot.
- Enjoy.

☐ **Nutritional facts:** Water, mineral and carbohydrate content is high

☐ **Calories:** 66 calories/ 100 g

Lamb with tomatoes

Ingredients:
- Lamb meat 500 grams
- Onion 2 chopped
- Ginger paste 1 tablespoon
- Tomato sauce half cup
- Salt as required

Method:
- Combine all ingredients in slow cooker.
- Cook till becomes soft.
- Enjoy.

☐ **Nutritional facts:** Vitamins, fat and carbohydrates
☐ **Calories:** 72 calories/ 100 g

Chapter 5- 10Super Gluten Free slow cooker recipes (Some additional recipes)

Spinach and turkey rice

Ingredients:
- Rice boiled 2 cups
- Spinach boiled half cup
- Turkey boiled 1 cup
- Chili sauce and salt as required

Method:
- Combine all ingredients except rice in slow cooker.
- Cook till hot.

☐ **Nutritional facts:** Water, mineral and carbohydrate content is high

☐ **Calories:** 40 calories/ 100 g

Chili cheese chicken mince

Ingredients:
- Chicken mince 200 grams
- Black pepper and salt as required
- Onion 2 chopped
- Oil 2 tablespoon

Method:
- Add all ingredients in to slow cooker and switch on the stove.
- Cook till mince becomes tender.

☐ **Nutritional facts:** Vitamins, fat and carbohydrates
☐ **Calories:** 33 calories/ 100 g

Spiced nuts

Ingredients:

- Nuts 1 cup roasted
- Oil 2 tablespoon
- Sugar a pinch
- Garlic paste 1 tablespoon
- Barbeque sauce as required

Method:

- Roast all nuts in slow cooker.
- Take out till cooked.

☐ **Nutritional facts:** Vitamins, fat and carbohydrates
☐ **Calories:** 63 calories/ 100 g

Turkey cabbage curry

Ingredients:

- Turkey half kg
- Cabbage chopped 1 cup
- Ginger paste 2 tablespoon
- Barbeque sauce 2 tablespoon
- Salt to taste
- Oil 2 tablespoon

Method:

- Add all ingredients in slew cooker.
- Cook till hot

☐ **Nutritional facts:** Minerals, carbohydrates and water content is high

☐ **Calories:**84 calories/ 100 g

Capsicum with mayonnaise

Ingredients:
- Mayonnaise 1 cup
- Capsicum 2 chopped
- Hot sauce and pepper 1 teaspoon

Method:
- Add all ingredients to slow cooker till hot.

☐ **Nutritional facts:** Minerals, carbohydrates and water content is high

☐ **Calories:**56 calories/ 100 g

Spinach potato cutlet

- Potato boiled and Spinach boiled 1 cup each
- Chili sauce and salt as required
- Corn flour to coat

Method:

- Combine all ingredients except corn flour.
- Make cutlets.
- Cook in slow cooker till hot.

☐ **Nutritional facts:** Water, mineral and carbohydrate content is high

☐ **Calories:** 54 calories/ 100 g

Sweet potatoes with apricots

Ingredients:

- Sweet potatoes 2 boiled
- Barbeque sauce 2 tablespoon
- Oil 2 tablespoon
- Sugar a pinch
- Apricots canned 1 cup

Method:

- Combine all ingredients in slow cooker.
- Cook till hot.

☐ **Nutritional facts:** Water, mineral and carbohydrate content is high

☐ **Calories:** 76 calories/ 100 g

Ginger Potato

Ingredients:
- Ginger paste 2 tablespoon
- Potato 2 boiled
- Spring onion 1 cup chopped
- Oil 2 tablespoon

Method:
- Add oil and all other ingredients in slow cooker.
- Cook till hot.
- Enjoy.

☐ **Nutritional facts:** Vitamins, fat and carbohydrates
☐ **Calories:** 98 calories/ 100 g

Potato cauliflower pie

Ingredients:
- Potato large 2 boiled
- Soy sauce 1 tablespoon
- Salt and pepper as required
- Cauliflower 1 cup roasted

Method:
- Combine potato with soy sauce
- Add oil in with other ingredients in slow cooker.
- Cook till complete.
- Enjoy.

☐ **Nutritional facts:** Water, mineral and carbohydrate content is high
☐ **Calories:** 90 calories/ 100 g

Red chili chicken pie

Ingredients:
- Chicken boneless 4
- Red chili paste 2 tablespoon
- Vinegar and soy sauce 2 teaspoon each
- Oil 3 tablespoon

Method:
- Add oil in slow cooker followed by rest of ingredients.
- Cook till hot.

☐ **Nutritional facts:** Vitamins, fat and carbohydrates
☐ **Calories:** 96 calories/ 100 g

Conclusion

Thank you again for downloading this book!

I am hoping that this book will help you to the maximum level in getting a wholesome knowledge of gluten free slow cooker recipes and the complete procedure of how to make them all. With the fact that mostly people are not aware of the gluten free recipes and how to cook them. I am also known as the fact that people are having a very little knowledge regarding it. So I have come out with this book to help you out in learning free and interesting gluten free recipes. I have started it with the very basic information regarding all recipes so that you must be aware of the fact that how it is made and what are the nutritional facts of it.

I have added all recipes in this book after getting so much experience. These recipes have been written step by step so that you can easily comprehend all the steps including for making perfect gluten free recipes. The categorization of recipes in this book has been done in such a way that you can easily go through different recipes of chicken, lamb and beef recipes. Every chapter have got sociality recipes which you will love. Step by step recipe making has also been added to avoid any confusion.

I am hopeful that my book of gluten free recipes would help all my readers in learning all the recipes easily in all aspect of gluten free recipes. This book will be surely beneficial for all the readers out there who want gluten free recipes.

Part 2

INTRODUCTION

What is Gluten?

Gluten, a Latin word meaning "glue", is a protein found in wheat that gives elasticity to dough, helping it to rise and keep its shape. Gluten is a combination of gliadin and glutenin: Gliadin is what enables bread to rise properly while glutenin is the major protein in wheat flour, making up 47% of the total protein content.

Common sources of gluten are barley (including malt, malt flavoring and malt vinegar), rye, triticale (a cross between wheat and rye) and wheat. Also on the list are bulgur, durum flour, farina, graham flour, kamut, semolina and spelt. Commercially, gluten is also found in foods such as beer, breads, cakes and pies, candies, cereals, cookies, crackers, croutons, some French fries, gravies, imitation meat and seafood, pastas, processed luncheon meats, some salad dressings, sauces including soya sauce, seasoned rice mixes, seasoned snack foods, such as potato and tortilla chips, soups and soup bases, and sauces, among others.

Gluten Sensitivity

Worldwide, gluten is a very common protein in most diets. Even so, about 1 in 133 people in developed nations have celiac disease, a genetic autoimmune disease that may cause the immune system to react adversely to the gliadin contained in gluten.[2] Celiac disease (also spelled Coeliac) is a disorder where the ingestion of gluten can lead to damage in the small intestine. This immune system attack can lead to damage on the villi, these small finger-like projections that protect the intestine and promote nutrient absorption[3]. When gluten attacks these villi, nutrients cannot be absorbed properly. The Celiac Disease Foundation adds that an estimated 2.5 million Americans are unaware that they have this disease.

Symptoms of Celiac Disease in adults and children include the following[4]:

Physical
- abdominal pain
- anaemia
- bone and joint defects such as arthritis and osteoporosis
- constipation
- delayed physical development
- dental problems
- diarrhoea
- fatigue
- headache
- infertility
- joint pain
- short stature

- thyroid problems
- vomiting
- weight loss

Mental and Behavioural
- Attention Deficit Hyperactivity Disorder (ADHD)
- depression
- delayed mental growth
- irritability
- lack of motivation

It is very important that Celiac Disease be diagnosed as early as possible because of the long term health problems associated with it[5]: These include:

- Autoimmune disease (thyroid problems, Type 1 diabetes, lupus, rheumatoid arthritis, and Sjögren's syndrome)
- Birth defects (in offspring)
- Delayed physical development
- Infertility
- Intestinal cancer
- Osteoporosis
- Miscarriage or infertility
- Seizures

Celiac Disease is diagnosed through several methodologies: (1) the tTG-IgA blood exam; (2) endoscopic biopsy; (3) gluten sensitivity test, used when people test negative for gluten antibodies but experience negative symptoms in response to eating gluten.

The Gluten-Free Lifestyle

Gluten-free diets were once not as popular as they are today, as they were only suggested for people suffering from Celiac Disease. However, with more research on the disease and the structures and dynamics of gluten, the impacts of gluten consumption have been explored more than ever. As a result, more and more people are choosing gluten-free diets because of the host of health benefits, and the many studies on the realities of gluten intolerance and wheat allergy, as well as gluten's indirect effect on peoples' long-term health and wellbeing. Recent research also points to gluten being at the root of obesity, with its consumption connected to hypothyroidism and an imbalance of hormones[6].

The health benefits of adopting a gluten-free diet far outweigh the feelings of withdrawal and the sacrifices people have to make at the start of their lifestyle change. However, the many benefits include the following:

- Decreased inflammation[7] and a reduction in a number of sensitivities proven to be sparked by the consumption of gluten. It is believed that more gluten-related sensitivities are yet to be proven.

- Consumption of fewer processed foods, thus more natural foods are enjoyed.

- Improved overall health[5] with a gluten free lifestyle. Some people experience weight loss because of an improved hormonal balance, and there are reduced health risks for conditions like diabetes. Others enjoy better skin, and an improved overall physical and mental performance.

However, it should be noted that people embarking on this lifestyle should proceed with care, since limiting their diet to gluten-free foods could also limit their nutrient intake. Important nutrients to keep in check are: iron, calcium, fiber, thiamin, riboflavin, niacin, and folate.

Stocking Up

An important list of what is safe to eat and what to avoid is highlighted below:

Allowed foods

- Fresh dairy products

- Fresh eggs
- Fresh meats, fish, and poultry
- Fruits and vegetables
- Legumes

The following grains can be substituted for gluten as long as they are kept in their fresh state or when processed in gluten-free environments and certified "gluten free."

- Amaranth
- Arrowroot
- Buckwheat
- Corn and cornmeal
- Flax
- Gluten-free flours (rice, soy, corn, potato, bean)
- Corn (hominy)
- Millet
- Quinoa
- Rice
- Sorghum
- Soy
- Tapioca
- Teff

Always avoid
___

- Barley (including malt, malt flavoring and malt vinegar)
- Bulgur

- Durum flour
- Farina
- Graham flour
- Kamut
- Oats, except certified gluten free (can be contaminated during the production process)
- Rye
- Semolina
- Spelt
- Triticale
- Wheat

Watch Out!

Take note of the following foods and only consume when labelled "gluten free":

- Candy
- Chips
- Processed meats such as ham, sausage, salami, seafood
- Wheat flour-based pastries, including breads, cakes, cereals, cookies, crackers, and pies
- Wheat flour-based pastas
- Sauces thickened with wheat flour, including gravy, salad dressings, soya sauce

Non-Food Products

It is important to check the labels of medicines and cosmetics, since many manufacturers use gluten as a filler. Also, some alcohol is distilled from grains that contain gluten and must be avoided.

Important Considerations

While there are many gluten free products available in the market, it is best to stick to natural products that are free of alteration and preservatives. For example, it is best to buy rice grains and not ready-to-eat rice packs, and fresh potatoes instead of powdered, frozen French fries, or potato chips.

Gluten-free substitutes for favorite recipes

Switching to gluten free does not have to mean you have to give up your favorite foods. Here is a list of gluten free substitutes for common recipes and ingredients[8]:

Ingredient	Gluten-Free Substitute
Breadcrumbs	Gluten-free oats, flax
Granola	Chopped nuts
Oatmeal	Gluten-free oats, grits
Roux	Corn starch and water, or potatoes
Soya sauce	Bragg's Liquid Aminos
Wheat flour	Corn, rice, potato, almond, coconut flour, black beans
Wheat	Zucchini, eggplant, rice

SNACK RECIPES

DIY Trail Mix

Yields about 4 1/4 cups
Preparation Time: 40 minutes

Ingredients:
1/3 cup pumpkin seeds
3/4 cup peanuts
2 cups millet
1/3 cup syrup sweetener (any kind)
3/4 tablespoon vanilla extract
3/4 teaspoon salt
3 egg whites

Directions:
1. Preheat the oven to 350ºF. Place a silicon baking sheet on the baking tray and set it aside.
2. In a mixing bowl, combine the millet, peanuts, and pumpkin seeds. Set aside.
3. Whisk together egg whites, sweetener, salt, and vanilla. Pour over nut mixture, and combine well.
4. Transfer the mix onto the baking sheet, and bake for 30 minutes.
5. Allow to cool before serving.

Apple Oatmeal Snacks

Servings: 10-12 bars
Preparation Time: 60 minutes

Ingredients:
2 ½ cups oats
¼ cup brown sugar
1 ½ teaspoons baking powder
1 ½ teaspoons nutmeg
Pinch salt
2 cups milk
4 eggs
1 apple, cut into small slices

Directions:
1. Preheat the oven to 350ºF. Grease a muffin pan with melted butter and set it aside.
2. In a bowl, mix together the oats, brown sugar, baking powder, nutmeg, and salt.
3. In a separate bowl, whisk together milk and egg.
4. Combine the wet and the dry ingredients, and whisk well. Fold in the apple pieces.
5. Fill each prepared muffin cup with the mixture. Bake for 35-45 minutes.

6. Let cool for 5 minutes before serving.

Homemade Granola

Servings: 6
Preparation Time: 50 minutes

Yields about 5 1/2 cups

Ingredients:
4 cups oats
2 tablespoons sunflower seeds
2 tablespoons pumpkin seeds
½ cup chopped peanuts
1 teaspoon cinnamon
1 teaspoon nutmeg
1 teaspoon salt
1 cup brown sugar
1/3 cup vegetable oil
1 teaspoon vanilla extract

Directions:
1. Preheat the oven to 375ºF and place the oven rack in the middle position.
2. In a bowl, mix all the ingredients.
3. Spread mixture on a rimmed baking sheet lined with parchment paper. Bake for 25 to 35 minutes until golden brown.

4. Let it cool for 5 minutes. Store the granola in an airtight container.

Fruit and Nut Yogurt

Servings: 1
Preparation Time: 5 minutes

Ingredients:
1 peach, pitted and halved
½ cup of vanilla yogurt (or any flavor you prefer)
1 tsp liquid honey
1 tablespoon chopped nuts like walnuts or pecans

Directions:
1. In a small bowl, mix together the yogurt and honey.
2. Add the peaches and combine well. Garnish with nuts and serve.

Fruity Greens Smoothie

Servings: 2
Preparation Time: 5 minutes

Ingredients:
1 cup baby spinach
2 tablespoons ground flax seed
1 pear
2 bananas
2 cups milk
1 tablespoon sugar

Directions:
1. In a blender, combine all ingredients.
2. Blend for about 2 minutes until smooth.
3. Serve cold

Chocolate Peppermint Milkshake

Servings: 1
Preparation Time: 5 minutes

Ingredients:

1 large banana
1 tablespoon cocoa
1/4 teaspoon peppermint syrup
2 teaspoons sugar
1 cup milk (any kind)

Directions:
1. In a blender, combine all ingredients.
2. Blend for about 2 minutes until smooth.
3. Serve cold

Spicy Spinach Chips Recipe

Servings: 2
Preparation Time: 35 minutes

Ingredients:
3 cups spinach
3 tablespoons olive oil
Kosher salt
1 pinch red crushed chili pepper flakes

Directions:
1. Preheat the oven to 350 ºF.
2. Rinse the spinach and dry with a paper towel. Remove large stems.
3. Toss the spinach and oil together. Do this gently until the leaves are well coated.
4. Arrange spinach leaves on a baking sheet
5. Sprinkle with salt and the crushed red chili flakes to taste.
6. Bake for 20-25 minutes.

Spiced Up Apple Cinnamon Chips

Servings: 6
Preparation Time: 140 minutes

Ingredients:
3 green apples, washed and cored
2 teaspoons cinnamon
1 teaspoon nutmeg
2 teaspoons sugar (white or brown)

Directions:
1. Preheat the oven to 200ºF. Line the baking tray with oven-friendly paper like parchment paper.
2. Slice the apples to 1/8th inch thickness with a mandolin slicer.
3. Mix together cinnamon, nutmeg, and sugar in a medium-size bowl.
4. Add apple slices to the spice mix. Stir to coat apples completely.
5. Arrange the apple slices in a single layer on a baking sheet and bake for 1 ½ to 2 hours.

Sweet Potato Fries

Servings: 2-3
Preparation Time: 40

Ingredients:
2 large sweet potatoes, washed
1 tablespoon brown sugar
2 tablespoons olive oil
Salt and pepper

Directions:
1. Preheat the oven to 375ºF
2. Slice sweet potatoes into long strips.
3. Coat with brown sugar, salt, and pepper.
4. Bakes for 25 to 30 minutes or till the fries turn golden brown and tender.

Roasted Yams

Servings: 4-5
Preparation Time: 55 minutes

Ingredients:
2 large yams (sweet potatoes)
2 tsp vegetable oil
1 tsp ground cumin

Salt

Directions:
1. Preheat the oven to 400ºF. Line baking sheet with foil.
2. Slice yams into thin rounds.
3. In a large mixing bowl, combine yams, oil, ground cumin and salt and mix gently.
4. Place yam slices on the baking sheet and roast for 35-45 minutes.

Squash Pie Shake

Servings: 1
Preparation Time: 5 minutes

Ingredients:
1 cup kale
2 cups milk (any kind)
1/2 cup cooked squash
2 teaspoons cinnamon
Sweetener (honey, sugar, agave, or any type preferred)
4-5 ice cubes

Directions:
1. In a blender, combine all ingredients.
2. Blend for about 2 minutes until smooth.

3. Serve cold.

Classic Spicy Homemade Popcorn

Servings: 2-4
Preparation Time: 5 minutes

Ingredients:
3 tablespoons butter
2 tablespoons vegetable oil
1 cup popcorn kernels
Salt and pepper
1 pinch or more of cayenne pepper
1 teaspoon sweet paprika

Directions:
1. Heat the butter and oil on a medium heat. Add the corn kernels, cover and let pop.
2. Place a heavy lid in such a manner that there is little space for the steam to escape.
3. The popping should start within 45 seconds,
4. Once the gap between pops is about 2 seconds, turn off the heat.
5. Season with cayenne pepper, paprika, and salt and pepper to taste.

Buttery Pumpkin Cake

Servings: 4-6
Preparation Time: 70 minutes

Ingredients:
1 cup butter, melted
2 cups brown sugar
2 cups pumpkin, cut into chunks
½ cup raisins
3 eggs
2 cups rice flour
2 tsp. cinnamon
¼ cup walnuts, chopped

Directions:
1. In a food processor, shred the pumpkin and set aside.
2. Preheat the oven to 325°F. Grease and line the bottom of a loaf pan with parchment paper.
3. Whisk butter and sugar in a bowl; add pumpkin and raisins. Mix well.
4. Add rice flour, cinnamon, nuts (reserving a few for the top) and combine.
5. Pour the batter into the loaf tin, sprinkle with remaining nuts, cinnamon and sugar

6. Bake for 55-60 minutes or until the cake is cooked through and a toothpick comes out clean when inserted in the middle.

Sugar and Spice Nuts

Servings: 2
Preparation Time: 5 minutes

Ingredients:
2 tablespoons brown sugar
1 tablespoon butter, melted
1 teaspoon cinnamon, ground
1 teaspoon cardamom, ground
2 tablespoons milk powder
1 cup of mixed nuts

Directions:
1. Combine brown sugar, melted butter, cinnamon, cardamom, milk powder, and mixed nuts in a bowl.
2. Microwave for 1 minute then cool to serve.

Greek-Style Hummus

Servings: 2 small bowls
Preparation Time: 10 minutes

Ingredients:
2 cloves garlic, minced
1 cup plain yogurt
1/2 cup fresh milk
1 teaspoon ground black pepper
1 teaspoon rosemary
1/2 cup garbanzo beans, boiled or canned
1/2 cup kidney beans, boiled or canned
2 teaspoons honey

Directions:
1. In a medium mixing bowl, mash the garbanzo beans, kidney beans, and garlic. For smoother consistency, use a food processor.
2. Add the yogurt, milk, black pepper, rosemary, and honey. Stir or pulse to combine.

Bruschetta

Servings: 6
Preparation Time: 10 minutes

Ingredients:

4 large tomatoes, chopped

2 tablespoons fresh rosemary, chopped (or 2 teaspoons dried)

2 tablespoons fresh oregano, chopped (or 2 teaspoons dried)

2 tablespoons fresh flat leaf parsley, chopped (or 2 teaspoons dried)

1 teaspoon black pepper

1 tablespoon olive oil

1/2 onion, finely chopped

1 garlic clove

Gluten-free country-style bread

Directions:

1. Mix together tomatoes, rosemary, oregano, parsley, black pepper, oil, and chopped onion thoroughly. Set aside.
2. Preheat the oven to 400ºF.
3. Slice the bread into thick slices. Place on a baking sheet and grill for 5-6 minutes, until golden brown.
4. Slice the garlic clove in half. Rub the garlic onto the grilled bread.
5. Place dollops of the tomato mixture on top of toasted gluten-free bread. Spread it and serve.

No-Bake Flax and Sesame Protein Bars

Servings: 8 bars
Preparation Time: 3 hours

Ingredients:
½ cup flax seeds
¼ cup sesame seeds
¼ cup raisins
½ cup mixed nuts
¼ cup low fat vanilla or plain yogurt
¼ cup honey

Directions:
1. Line the bottom and sides of a 9-inch loaf pan with parchment. Place the flax seeds, raisins, mixed nuts, yogurt, and honey in a food processor. Pulse until well combined, just a few seconds.
2. Spread the mixture in the baking pan and refrigerate for 2-3 hours, or until set.
3. Cut into bars and serve.

BREAKFAST RECIPES

Eggs and Everything Nice Toast Cups

Servings: 8
Preparation Time: 50 minutes

Ingredients:
Butter
8 slices gluten-free bread
8 slices gluten-free ham
8 eggs
Salt and pepper

Directions:
1. Preheat the oven to 375ºF.
2. Grease the muffin cups with melted butter. Flatten bread with a rolling pin, a clean bottle, or your hand. Place the flattened bread into each cup.
3. In a hot pan, fry the ham pieces till they are lightly browned.
4. Place one slice of ham in the muffin cup, on top of the flattened bread, then break an egg over it. Season with salt and pepper.
5. Bake for 25-30 minutes.
6. Serve hot.

Corn and Cheese Omelet

Servings: 2
Preparation Time: 15 minutes

Ingredients:
2 tablespoons olive oil
4 potatoes, peeled and shredded
1/2 cup corn (fresh or canned)
3 eggs, lightly beaten
¼ cup milk (2% or whole milk)
Salt and pepper
½ cup cheddar cheese, grated

Direction:
1. In a medium mixing bowl, beat eggs and milk until the mixture is well combined. Season to taste with salt and pepper.
2. Heat olive oil in a large skillet over medium-high heat.
3. Fry potatoes until almost cooked, about 4-5 minutes.
4. Add corn, and stir. Carefully pour in the egg and milk mixture.
5. Cook until the eggs are set.
6. Add the grated cheese.
7. Flip half of the omelet over the other half, cook for 1-2 minutes more until the cheese is well melted.
8. Serve immediately.

Kale and Tomato Omelet

Servings: 2
Preparation Time: 10 minutes

Ingredients:
2 tablespoons vegetable oil
1 cup kale leaves, chopped
3 eggs
1/4 cup tomatoes, chopped
1/4 cup cheddar cheese, grated

Directions:
1. Stir fry the kale for 3-4 minutes. Add the tomatoes and sauté briefly.
2. In a medium mixing bowl, beat the eggs. Gently stir in the kale mixture.
3. Heat oil in a pan, pour in the eggs and kale mixture and spread evenly.
4. When bottom is set, flip it over and cook for another minute. When eggs cooked from both side, grate the cheese and fold the omelet, so the cheese melts.
5. Serve hot.

Strawberries and Hot Grits

Servings: 2
Preparation Time: 10 minutes

Ingredients:
3/4 cup grits, uncooked
3 cups milk (any kind)
1/4 cup sugar
1/4 cup strawberries
1/4 cup peanuts

Directions:
1. Boil milk in a saucepan on medium-high heat for 5 minutes. Lower the heat to medium-low, add the grits and sugar, and stir until the mixture thickens.
2. Add strawberries and nuts; and stir gently for 2-3 minutes.
3. Serve hot.

Yummy Bagels

Servings: 4
Preparation Time: 80 minutes

Ingredients:
2 teaspoons dry yeast
2 cups water
5 cups potato flour

4 tablespoons sugar
1 teaspoon salt
2 quarts boiling water
3 teaspoons oil (any type preferred)

Directions:
1. In a bowl, dissolve yeast in water.
2. Mix the flour, sugar, and salt into the yeast mixture, mix until it forms a dough.
3. Divide the dough into four equal pieces. On a floured working surface, roll long strips and form into a bagel shape. Cover with a clean, damp kitchen towel and allow to rise for 35-45 minutes.
4. Preheat the oven to 300ºF.
5. Boil water in a large stock pot. Place bagels in boiling water for 40 seconds. Remove the bagels from water and then place them on a baking sheet greased with oil.
6. Bake for 20 minutes.

Happy Breakfast Burrito

Servings: 2
Preparation Time: 5 minutes

Ingredients:
3 eggs

1/2 green bell pepper, diced
1/2 cup cheddar cheese, grated
2 teaspoons vegetable oil
Rice tortillas
Salt and pepper
Tomatoes, diced

Directions:
1. Beat eggs in a mixing bowl. Stir in green bell pepper, salt, and pepper.
2. Heat the oil in a large skillet on medium-high. Add the egg mixture when the oil is hot. Fry until the edges are golden.
3. Add cheese on half of the omelet. Flip the other side over, and cook until the cheese melts.
4. Remove from heat
5. Wrap eggs in the rice tortillas.
6. Top with diced tomatoes

Spiced Up Eggs

Servings: 4
Preparation Time: 15 minutes

Ingredients:
3 tablespoons olive oil
½ green bell pepper, diced

½ red bell pepper, diced
½ small yellow onion, diced
4 large tomatoes, the centers scooped out to create a cup
1 tablespoon hot sauce
5 eggs
½ cup plain yogurt
1 garlic clove, minced

Directions:
1. Heat the oil in a large skillet on medium-high heat.
2. Stir fry both green and red peppers with onions for 2 minutes, until fragrant and tender.
3. Add garlic, and continue cooking for 1 minute.
4. Beat the eggs, and add to the skillet. Scramble the eggs with the vegetables for 1-2 minutes, or until set. Remove from heat and reserve.
5. 'Mix the yogurt with the hot sauce. Stir well.
6. Place cooked eggs inside the tomatoes.
7. Top with the spicy yogurt.

Spanish Omelet

Servings: 3
Preparation Time: 7 to 10 minutes

Ingredients:

1 cup potatoes, diced
2 tablespoons butter
1 onion, sliced
1 red bell pepper, chopped
6 eggs
Parsley, chopped

Directions:
1. Heat butter in a pan over medium heat. Add the potatoes and stir fry for 4-5 minutes. Add the onion and pepper and cook for 1 or 2 minutes until tender.
2. Beat the eggs in a bowl.
3. Add the beaten egg to the vegetables and spread the egg mix evenly in the pan.
4. Let the egg set until well cooked, about 2-3 minutes.
5. Serve hot and garnish with parsley.

LUNCH RECIPES

Savory Bean and Potato Soup

Servings: 4-5
Preparation Time: 25 minutes

Ingredients:
1 cup potatoes, chopped
1 cup carrots, chopped
½ cup canned black beans, drained and rinsed
½ cup canned kidney beans, drained and rinsed
1 red bell pepper, chopped
1 green bell pepper, chopped
2 cloves garlic, minced
2 tablespoons fresh rosemary, chopped
2 tablespoons fresh oregano, chopped
10 cups of broth (any kind)
Salt and pepper

Directions:
1. In a large stock pot, bring the broth to a boil. Add the chopped potatoes, carrots, red bell pepper, green bell pepper, garlic, rosemary and oregano. Cook until tender, about 15 minutes. Add the beans and heat through.
2. Season with salt and pepper.
3. Mix well and serve hot.

Cheesy Asparagus Soup

Servings: 3
Preparation Time: 20 minutes

Ingredients:
1 cup carrots, peeled and chopped
2 cups asparagus, chopped
1 teaspoon of cumin
1 teaspoon of black pepper
½ cup cheddar cheese, grated
5 cups of broth (any type preferred)
Dash of salt

Directions:
1. Bring the broth to a boil, and add the carrots, asparagus and cumin. Simmer for about 10 minutes.
2. Remove from heat, and allow to cool until you can place your hand on the side of the pot.
3. Add cheddar cheese, black pepper and dash of salt. Stir until the cheese melts.
4. You can add more grated cheddar cheese on top before serving. (optional)

Tomato and Grape Salad

Servings: 2
Preparation Time: 5 minutes

Ingredients:
1 cup table grapes
1 cup tomatoes, chopped
½ cup lemon juice
1 teaspoon ground black pepper
1 tablespoon oregano
1 tablespoon rosemary
2 tablespoons olive oil
1 tablespoon balsamic vinegar
Salt
Gluten-free bread
1 tablespoon parmesan cheese, grated

Directions:
1. Toss the grapes, tomatoes, lemon juice, black pepper, oregano, rosemary, olive oil, balsamic vinegar, and salt in a big bowl.
2. Top with parmesan cheese, and serve with gluten-free bread.

Tomato Nacho Soup

Servings: 6
Preparation Time: 20 minutes

Ingredients:
1 15 oz. can stewed tomatoes
½ cup onions, chopped
2 or 3 cloves garlic, minced
2 tablespoons vegetable oil
½ cup cheddar cheese, grated
½ cup tomato paste
½ cup tomato sauce
1 tablespoon oregano
1 tablespoon rosemary
4 cups chicken or vegetable broth
Salt and pepper
1 cup corn nachos (gluten-free), crushed

Directions:
1. Heat oil in a pan and sauté the onions and garlic
2. Add broth, stewed tomatoes, tomato paste, tomato sauce, oregano and rosemary. Mix well and let it simmer for 10-12 minutes.
3. Remove from heat and allow to cool slightly. Add grated cheddar cheese, and season with salt and pepper.
4. Add crushed nachos to the soup before serving.

Coconut and Squash Soup

Servings: 4
Preparation Time: 15 minutes

Ingredients:
2 tablespoons olive oil
½ onion, chopped
½ cup asparagus, chopped
2 cups zucchini, chopped
2 teaspoons ground turmeric
5 cups of broth (any kind)
¾ cup coconut milk
Salt and pepper

Directions:
1. Heat oil in a pan and sauté chopped onions for 1 minute. Add asparagus, squash, zucchini, ground turmeric and coconut milk.
2. Add the broth and simmer for 8-10 minutes.
3. Season with salt and pepper before serving.

Chili and Corn Bread

Servings: 6
Preparation Time: 55 minutes

Ingredients:

2 teaspoons vegetable oil

1 pound ground chicken

1 yellow onion, chopped

1 cup tomatoes, diced

1 15 oz. can of kidney beans, drained

1 tablespoon minced garlic

2 tablespoons chili powder

1 teaspoon parsley, chopped

1 teaspoon ground cumin

1 teaspoon salt

½ teaspoon ground black pepper

1½ cups chicken broth

1 tablespoon tomato paste

Directions:

1. Heat oil in a large non-stick pan and sauté the ground chicken for 20-25 minutes on low heat.
2. Add the onion, tomatoes, kidney beans, and garlic and cook for 2-3 minutes.
3. Add broth and tomato paste. Stir well to mix all the ingredients together.
4. Season with chili powder, parsley, ground cumin, salt, and pepper. Bring to a boil and reduce heat to medium-low and let simmer uncovered until reduced, about 20-30 minutes. Serve with cornbread, recipe below.

Buttermilk Cornbread

Servings: 6
Preparation time: 40 minutes

Ingredients:

2 cups buttermilk
1 cup cornmeal
1 teaspoon baking powder
½ teaspoon baking soda
1 cup gluten-free flour, all purpose
2 tablespoons white sugar
2 eggs
3 tablespoons butter

Directions:
1. Preheat the oven to 375°F.
2. Add the butter to a 10" cast iron skillet, and place it in the oven while you make the batter.
3. In a large bowl, whisk together the flour, baking soda, and baking powder. Add the cornmeal and mix until the ingredients are well blended.
4. In a separate bowl, whisk together the eggs and buttermilk. Add the sugar, and blend until the sugar is dissolved.
5. Remove the cast iron skillet from the oven, and tilt the skillet until it is completely coated in butter.
6. Pour the remaining butter into the egg mixture.

7. Add the wet ingredients to the dry, and mix until the batter is smooth.
8. Pour the batter into the skillet, and place in the oven.
9. Bake for 25 to 30 minutes or until the cornbread golden brown and springs back when pressed.
10. Serve warm on its own or with another dish.

Taco Salad

Servings: 6 to 8
Preparation Time: 40 minutes

Ingredients:
1½ pounds ground chicken
1 red bell pepper, diced
2 tablespoons gluten-free taco seasoning
¾ cup water
2 cups lettuce, shredded
½ cup tomato, diced
1 piece avocado, chopped
Salt and pepper
Corn chips

Directions:

1. In a large skillet, heat oil on medium heat, and sauté ground chicken for 25 minutes, until well cooked. Stir occasionally.
2. Add taco seasoning and water. Mix well. Reduce heat to medium-low and simmer until all the liquids have evaporated. Remove from heat.
3. Add red bell pepper, avocado, and tomato and mix well. Season with salt and pepper.
4. While the chicken is cooking, prepare the vegetables.
5. Place the lettuce in a large bowl. Spoon chicken, tomato and avocado on top.
6. Serve with corn chips.

Kale Pancakes

Servings: 4
Preparation Time: 30 minutes

Ingredients:
2 cups kale, chopped
½ cup red bell pepper, diced
¼ cup onion, chopped
2 tablespoons garlic, minced
1 tablespoon fresh ginger, grated
1 cup potato flour
½ cup chicken broth

½ teaspoon baking soda
1 tablespoon Dijon mustard
1 tablespoon fresh ginger, grated
Salt and pepper
Vegetable oil for frying
Sour cream and fresh chopped chives, for topping

Directions:
1. Heat about 2 tablespoons of vegetable oil in a large skillet. Sauté the onions, ginger, and garlic for 1-2 minutes until fragrant and tender.
2. Add kale and pepper. Stir-fry for 3-5 minutes until the kale is tender. Remove from heat and drain the vegetables, trying to get out most of the liquids.
3. In a mixing bowl, combine potato flour, chicken broth, baking soda, and mustard.
4. Mix well. Add the vegetables to the batter. Stir to coat.
5. Return the skillet to medium heat, and heat some oil.
6. Add about ¼ cup of the batter and fry on one side until the edges are crisp and golden. Flip over and cook for about 1 minute. Place on a hot plate.
7. Repeat until all the batter is used. Keep the pancakes warm by covering the plate with foil.
8. Serve with a dollop of sour cream and sprinkle chives on top

Tuna Bagels

Servings: 2
Preparation Time: 5 minutes

Ingredients:
1 cup canned tuna drained
Gluten-free bagel
Cream cheese

Directions:
1. Mix cream cheese and tuna in a bowl.
2. Top bagel with the mixture and serve.

Greek Toast

Servings: 1
Preparation Time: 5 minutes

Ingredients:
½ cup tomato, diced
Parsley, chopped
Cheddar cheese, grated
Gluten-free bread
2 teaspoons balsamic vinegar
2 teaspoons sesame oil

1. Slightly grease 2 slices of bread (one side of each bread) with balsamic vinegar and sesame oil. Place in toaster oven for 2 minutes.
2. Remove the toasted bread to a cutting board, greased side down. Place the diced tomato, parsley, and cheddar cheese on one slice, and layer the other slice on top to form a sandwich.

Spicy Tuna Salad

Servings: 2
Preparation Time: 5 minutes

Ingredients:
1 cup spicy tuna
½ onion, chopped
2 teaspoons fresh parsley, chopped
1 teaspoon minced garlic
½ cup mayonnaise
¼ teaspoon pepper
2 teaspoons chili powder
½ cup tomato, diced
3 cups iceberg lettuce
½ cup carrot, shredded

Directions:

1. Combine spicy tuna, onion, parsley, garlic, mayonnaise, pepper, chili pepper and tomato.
2. In another bowl, form a layer of iceberg lettuce and carrot.
3. Put the tuna mix on the lettuce and carrot bed and serve.

Chicken and Turkey Sandwich

Servings: 2
Preparation Time: 25 minutes

Ingredients:
4 slices gluten-free bread
2 slices deli smoked turkey
½ cup ground chicken (cooked)
4 butter lettuce leaves
2 slices red tomato
Honey Dijon mustard

Directions:
1. Place the turkey slice, a spoonful of ground chicken, lettuce, and tomato between 2 slices of gluten-free bread.
2. Top with mustard and serve.

Peanut and Rice Salad

Servings: 2
Preparation Time: 25 minutes

Ingredients:
½ cup cooked rice
½ cup carrots, shredded
½ cup tomatoes, diced
½ cup cheddar cheese, diced
¼ cup peanuts, ground
3 cups mixed baby greens
Salt and pepper

Directions:
1. Combine the cooked rice, carrots, tomatoes, cheddar cheese, and peanuts in a bowl
2. Whisk the olive oil, lemon juice, mustard, and honey until well combined.
3. Pour the dressing over the rice mixture. Stir to coat well.
4. Serve the rice on a bed of lettuce. Sprinkle with salt and pepper.

Pistachio Salad

Servings: 2
Preparation Time: 10 minutes

Ingredients:
3 teaspoons olive oil
2 teaspoons turmeric, ground
1 lemon, juiced
1 tablespoon honey
1 tablespoon fresh mint, chopped
1 cup kale, chopped
1 cup spinach
1 cup pistachios, shelled
½ cup peanuts, ground

Directions:
1. In a skillet over medium-high heat, sauté the pistachios and peanuts until slightly brown. Remove from heat and place in a mixing bowl.
2. Mix in turmeric, lemon, honey, mint, spinach, and kale.
3. Combine nuts and the kale mixture. Stir to coat, and serve.

Simple Chicken Rice Noodles

Servings: 4
Preparation Time: 25 minutes

Ingredients:
1 pound rice noodles
2 tablespoons canola oil, separated
1 cup green beans, trimmed and chopped
1 cup green cabbage, shredded
½ yellow onion, thinly sliced
1 carrot, shredded
2 cloves garlic, minced
2-3 tablespoons gluten-free soya sauce
1 cup cooked chicken breast, shredded
1-2 teaspoons red chili crushed pepper flakes (optional)

Directions:
1. Cook rice noodles as per instructions on the package and set aside.
2. In a large skillet or a wok, heat the oil on medium-high heat. Sauté onions and garlic for 1-2 minutes until tender.
3. Reduce the heat to medium-low. Add 1 tablespoon of oil. Add green beans, cabbage and carrot to the skillet. Sauté for 3-4 minutes on medium-low heat, until tender.
4. Add the chicken and heat for 1-3 minutes until heated through.
5. Add the cooked noodles, and enough soya sauce to coat all the ingredients. Cook for 1-3 minutes until

all the ingredients are well mixed and heated through.
6. Add pepper flakes, if you want some heat to your dish. Stir well.
7. Remove from heat and serve.

Quinoa, Nuts and Spices

Servings: 2
Preparation Time: 10 minutes

Ingredients:
2 tablespoons olive oil
2 bay leaves
1 teaspoon cumin
2 cups cooked quinoa
1 cup peanuts or cashews, chopped
½ cup cheddar cheese, grated
1 tablespoon fresh parsley, chopped
Salt and pepper

Directions:
1. Heat oil in a large skillet on medium-high heat, and sauté the bay leaves, cumin, quinoa, and nuts.
2. Season with salt and pepper
3. Garnish with the chopped parsley, cheddar cheese.
4. Remove bay leaves before serving.

Shrimp Salad

Servings: 4
Preparation Time: 20 minutes

Ingredients
2 carrots, diced
1 cup cauliflower florets, chopped
1 green bell pepper, diced
12 medium-sized shrimps, cooked
¼ cup freshly squeezed lemon juice
4 tablespoons sunflower oil
2 teaspoons Dijon mustard
½ cup tomatoes, diced
1 cup seedless green grapes, halved

Directions:
1. Mix together carrots, cauliflower, bell pepper, shrimps, lemon juice, sunflower oil, and mustard.
2. Top with tomatoes and grapes and serve.

Salmon and Asparagus Salad

Servings: 2
Preparation Time: 10 minutes

Ingredients:

20 asparagus spears
¾ cup salmon flakes
1 15 oz. can of black beans, rinsed
½ small yellow onion, diced
4 tablespoons olive oil
2 tablespoons balsamic vinegar
Salt and freshly ground black pepper

Directions:

1. Prepare a large bowl with ice cubes and very cold water. Set aside.
2. Steam the asparagus spears for 3-4 minutes in a double boiler, until just tender. Remove from heat and plunge the asparagus in the prepared bowl for 4-5 minutes, to stop the cooking process and keep asparagus' bright green color.
3. Chop the asparagus in bite-size pieces.
4. In a mixing bowl, combine the asparagus, black beans, onion, olive oil, and vinegar.
5. Stir in the salmon.
6. Serve the salad cold.

Creamy Beans and Potato Salad

Servings: 2
Preparation Time: 15 minutes

Ingredients:

1 15 oz. can pinto beans, rinsed
1 teaspoon chili powder
½ cup cucumber, diced
1 large French shallot, diced
1 tablespoon fresh parsley, chopped
3 large potatoes, cooked and diced
Salt and pepper
¼ cup Greek plain yogurt
2 tablespoons mayonnaise
1 tablespoon apple cider vinegar
1 teaspoon Dijon mustard
1 teaspoon fresh dill, chopped
1 teaspoon sweet relish

Directions:

1. In a salad bowl, mix the beans, chili powder, cucumber, shallot, parsley, and potatoes. Season with salt and pepper.
2. In a small mixing bowl, whisk the Greek yogurt, mayonnaise, apple cider vinegar, mustard, Dill, and relish.
3. Add the dressing to the potato mixture. Stir to coat all the ingredients.
4. Refrigerate 30 minutes before serving.

Watercress Rice Meal

Servings: 2
Preparation Time: 20 minutes

Ingredients:

2 eggs
1 onion, diced
2 tablespoons olive oil
2 cups watercress, chopped
1 cup milk
½ cup feta cheese
1 cup cooked rice

Directions:

1. Whisk the eggs, onion, watercress, milk, and feta cheese together.
2. Heat the oil in a wok on medium-high heat. Fry the egg mixture for 3-4 minutes.
3. Add rice and stir fry for another 1-2 minutes until the rice is hot.
4. Serve hot,

Beans and Greens Cream Soup

Servings: 2-4
Preparation Time: 25 minutes

Ingredients:

1 15 oz. can of red kidney beans, rinsed

½ onion, diced

2 cloves garlic, minced

¼ cup freshly squeezed lemon juice

1 cup green cabbage, shredded

1 zucchini, diced

1 cup kale, chopped

1 cup broccoli florets

1 cup spinach, chopped

1 tablespoon fresh parsley, chopped

4 cups chicken or vegetable broth

½ cup heavy cream

Salt and pepper

Directions:

1. In a large saucepan, heat the olive oil on medium-high heat. Sauté the onions and garlic for 1-2 minutes until tender.
2. Add lemon juice, cabbage, kale, broccoli, spinach, parsley, and broth.
3. Simmer the soup on medium heat for 8-10 minutes until all the vegetables are fork tender.
4. Season it with salt and pepper. Add kidney beans and cream. Cook for 2-3 minutes more.
5. With a submersible hand-held blender or food processor, purée the soup.
6. Serve hot.

Chicken Green Soup

Servings: 4
Preparation Time: 25 minutes

Ingredients:
2 tablespoons olive oil
1 onion, diced
1 garlic clove, minced
1 cup black beans, rinsed
2 cups kale, chopped
2 cups spinach, chopped
1 tomato, chopped
2 teaspoons ground turmeric
2 teaspoons paprika
1 cup cooked chicken, cubed
4 cups chicken or vegetable broth
1 tablespoon fresh parsley, chopped
Salt and pepper

Directions:
1. Heat the oil in a stock pot or soup kettle, and fry the onion and garlic for 1-2 minutes until tender. Add kale, spinach, and tomato. Sauté for about 2-3 minutes until kale is tender.
2. Add in the broth, chicken, black beans, ground turmeric, and paprika.
3. Season with salt and pepper

4. Bring to a boil on high heat. Reduce heat to medium-low and simmer for about 10-12 minutes.
5. Garnish with chopped parsley before serving.

Southern Californian Stew

Servings: 5
Preparation Time: 30 minutes

Ingredients:
1 cup dry mongo beans, rinsed
2 tablespoons vegetable oil
2 potatoes, diced
1 carrots, diced
1 cup green cabbage, shredded
½ red bell pepper, diced
½ green bell pepper, diced
2 teaspoons chili powder
½ onion, diced
¼ cup liquid honey
5 cups chicken or vegetable broth
Salt and pepper

Directions:
1. Bring water to a boil in a saucepan on high heat. Add mongo beans and cook for 10-15 minutes. Take care not to overcook the beans, as they will become mushy.
2. Heat the oil in a large skillet. Sauté the onions for 1-2 minutes until tender. Add potatoes, carrots, cabbage, red bell pepper, green bell pepper, chili

powder, and onion. Fry on medium-low heat for 5-6 minutes until the vegetables are tender.
3. Add the mongo beans to the sautéed vegetables and mix well.
4. Add the broth and honey. Bring to a boil on high heat, then reduce heat to medium and simmer for 10-12 minutes.
5. Season with salt and pepper before serving.

Asian Vegetable Stew

Servings: 2
Preparation Time: 25 minutes

Ingredients:
½ cup gluten-free soya sauce
½   cup   brown   sugar
2 tablespoons grape seed oil
1 onion, chopped
3 garlic cloves, minced
1 cup spinach, chopped
1 cup snow peas, trimmed and sliced
1 small can bamboo shoots, rinsed and drained
1 cup Chinese cabbage, chopped
2 cups chicken or vegetable broth
½ cup corn, frozen or canned
Salt and pepper

1 teaspoon of ground cumin

Directions:
1. Heat the oil in a wok on high heat, and sauté onion and garlic for 1-2 minutes until tender.
2. Add the spinach, Chinese cabbage, snow peas, and bamboo shoots. Sauté for 2-3 minutes.
3. Add soya sauce and brown sugar, and mix well for 3-5 more minutes.
4. Add broth and corn, and then simmer for 10-12 minutes.
5. Add a teaspoon of cumin and mix well.
6. Season with salt and pepper before serving

Fruit and Vegetable Stir-Fry

Servings: 2
Preparation Time: 15 minutes

Ingredients:
2 tablespoons canola oil
1 clove garlic, minced
¼ cup onion, chopped
1 cup spinach, chopped
1 cup red cabbage, shredded
1 cup apple, peeled, cored, and chopped
2 tablespoons raisins

1 teaspoon cardamom
1 teaspoon cinnamon
1 cup cooked brown rice

Directions:
1. Heat the oil in a sauté pan and fry garlic and onion for 1-2 minutes, until tender.
2. Add cabbage and sauté for 3-4 minutes before adding spinach, apple, raisins, cardamom, and cinnamon. Sauté until the cinnamon and cardamom become aromatic and all vegetables fork tender, about 3-4 minutes.
3. Place brown rice in 2 serving bowls. Top with stir-fry mixture.

DINNER RECIPES

Meaty Baked Lasagna

Servings: 4
Preparation Time: 1 hour 45 minutes

Ingredients:
1 package of gluten-free lasagna pasta, ready to use
2 tablespoons olive oil
2 pounds ground beef
1 large yellow onion, chopped
3 cloves garlic, minced
2 large cans of chopped Italian tomatoes
1 small can of tomato paste
¼ cup fresh basil, chopped2 teaspoons dried oregano
2 bay leaves
1 pinch crushed red chili flakes
3 cups mozzarella cheese, shredded

Directions:
1. Heat some oil in a large saucepan over medium heat. Sauté the onions for 1-2 minutes until tender and fragrant. Add the garlic. Brown the ground beef until cooked, about 6-7 minutes, and drain the fat. Add, tomatoes, tomato sauce, tomato paste, basil, and chili flakes. Reduce heat to low and let the sauce simmer, uncovered, for 45 minutes to an hour.

2. Preheat the oven to 350ºF and place oven rack in the middle position.
3. Spread 1/3 of the sauce in a lasagna baking dish. Spread 1/3 of the mozzarella cheese over the sauce. Place a single layer of the gluten-free lasagna pasta on top to cover the sauce and cheese mix. Top with 1/3 of the meat sauce. Add 1/3 of the shredded mozzarella. Cover again with lasagna. Pour the remaining sauce on top. Finish by adding the remaining mozzarella.
4. Cover the lasagna with aluminum foil (or the baking dish lid if it has one). Place in the oven and bake for 40 minutes. Remove the foil and continue baking for another 10 minutes or until the cheese is golden and the edges of the lasagna are bubbly and golden brown.

Baked Ziti Pasta

Serves 6
Preparation: 75 minutes

Ingredients
2 tablespoons olive oil
½ cup onion, chopped
1 cup mushrooms, sliced
1 cup green bell pepper, chopped

2 cloves garlic, minced
1 cup water
¼ cup fresh Italian parsley, chopped
Sea salt and freshly ground black pepper
½ teaspoon dried oregano
½ teaspoon dried basil
½ teaspoon dried thyme
2 14-oz. cans whole tomatoes; reserve liquid and chop
1 6-oz. can tomato paste
3 cups gluten-free ziti pasta
¾ cup fresh parmesan cheese, grated
¾ cup mozzarella cheese, shredded

Directions:
1. Cook gluten-free pasta according to package directions.
2. Add olive oil to a skillet over medium heat. Add onion, mushrooms, bell pepper and garlic. Sauté until tender, about 3-4 minutes.
3. Preheat the oven to 375ºF.
4. In a large pot combine water, parsley, seasonings, tomatoes, and tomato paste. Bring to a boil; reduce heat and simmer about 20 minutes. Remove from heat and cool lightly.
5. When cooled, combine sauce, onion mixture, ziti, and about half of each of the cheeses in a large mixing bowl. Stir to blend. Pour into a 9 x 13" baking dish. Cover and bake in the oven for 35-40 minutes.
6. Remove from oven, uncover and sprinkle with remaining half of cheeses. Broil in the oven for 1-2

minutes until the cheese is melted and golden brown, about 5 minutes.

Surprise Chicken and Eggs

Servings: 2-4
Preparation Time: 40 minutes

Ingredients:
1 pound boneless chicken breast
1 tablespoon olive oil
1 cup mushrooms, sliced
1 cup milk
2 eggs
1 spring of fresh rosemary
3 cloves garlic, minced
½ cup cheddar cheese, shredded
Salt and pepper

Directions:
1. Preheat the oven to 350ºF
2. Place chicken in a roasting pan. Brush with olive oil and season with salt and pepper. Roast the chicken, together with the rosemary and garlic, for 20-25 minutes until the chicken is cooked through.
3. Add 1 tablespoon of olive oil to a large skillet and heat over medium-high heat. Add mushrooms and sauté for 2-3 minutes. Remove from heat and reserve.

4. Whisk together milk and eggs in a small mixing bowl. Add the egg mixture to the skillet and scramble the eggs over medium-high heat, about 2-3 minutes. Season with salt and pepper and add the cheese. Remove from heat when the eggs are cooked, and reserve.
5. When ready to serve, divide the scrambled eggs onto serving plates. Slice the chicken into strips and arrange it on top of the eggs.

Beef Sausage Stew

Servings: 6 to 8
Preparation Time: 1 hour

Ingredients:
10 beef sausages
2 tablespoons olive oil
1 carrot, chopped
2 potatoes, chopped
¼ small green cabbage, shredded
1 onion, diced
1 tablespoon fresh parsley, chopped
1 15 oz. can stewed tomatoes
8 cups beef broth
2 teaspoons chili powder
Salt and pepper

Directions:

1. In a large saucepan, heat the olive oil on medium-high heat. Sauté the onions for 1-2 minutes until tender.
2. Add the sausage and fry for 5-6 minutes until cooked.
3. Add carrot, potatoes, cabbage, parsley, and tomatoes. Sauté for 4-5 minutes.
4. Add the chili powder and stir to coat.
5. Pour the broth in the mix and simmer for 30 minutes.
6. Taste and season with salt and pepper to taste before serving.

Steak with a Asparagus and Potato Hash

Servings: 3
Preparation Time: 25 minutes

Ingredients:

3 sirloin steaks, 4-6 oz. each
1 teaspoon garlic powder
1-2 teaspoons Montreal steak spice
2 tablespoons olive oil
2 red potatoes, cut in small cubes
1 clove garlic, minced

Salt and pepper
1 tablespoon fresh parsley, chopped
1 tablespoon fresh basil, chopped
1 tablespoon fresh thyme, chopped
20 fresh asparagus spears, trimmed and chopped
¼ cup lemon, squeezed

Directions:

1. Season the steaks generously with garlic powder and steak spice. Let the steak rest for 10-15 minutes before cooking. Grill steaks on the barbecue or under the oven broiler to desired doneness. Cover with foil and set aside.
2. Add the olive oil to a large skillet, and set the heat to medium-high. Sauté the onion and garlic for 1-2 minutes, until tender.
3. Lower the heat to medium. Add potatoes, parsley, basil, thyme, and asparagus and lemon juice. Season with salt and pepper. Stir-fry for about 5-6 minutes until the potatoes and asparagus are fork tender. Remove from heat.
4. To serve, top the steaks with the hash. Season with salt and pepper if desired.

Norwegian-Style Salmon Fillets

Servings: 4

Preparation Time: 80

Ingredients:
4 salmon fillets of even size
1 tablespoon olive oil
Salt and pepper
1 lime, juiced
2 tablespoons butter, melted
1 cup watercress
1 cup spinach
2 tablespoons dry white wine

Directions:
1. In a mixing bowl, combine oil butter, lime juice, and a sprinkle of salt and pepper, and white wine.
2. Place the salmon fillets in the marinade and refrigerate one hour.
3. Place this preparation in a preheated oven at 350ºF for 10 minutes.
4. Heat some oil in a pan and sauté the watercress with salt and pepper.
5. Serve baked salmon fillets with sautéed watercress.

Rosemary Turkey

Servings: 3
Preparation Time: 50 minutes

Ingredients:
1 pound turkey meat
1 ½ tablespoons of oil (any type preferred)
2 pieces of onion, chopped
3 pieces of garlic, mashed
5 teaspoons of rosemary, roughly chopped
Salt and pepper

Directions:
6. Preheat the oven to 350ºF
1. Roast turkey for 30-40 minutes.
2. Sauté the onion, garlic, rosemary and season it with salt and pepper.
3. Serve the onion mix on a plate and top the roasted turkey over it.

Mac & Cheese

Servings: 3
Preparation Time: 50 minutes

Ingredients:
3 cups gluten-free macaroni, cooked
½ cup butter
1 teaspoon cumin
1 small onion, chopped

1 clove garlic, minced
2 cups milk
2 cups cheddar cheese, grated
Salt and pepper

Directions:
1. Preheat the oven to 375 ºF.
2. Heat the butter and mix the chopped onion, mashed garlic, salt and pepper, cumin, and milk and let it simmer for 5 minutes.
3. Pour this mix over the boiled macaroni pasta and stir in the grated cheese. Bake for 30-40 minutes.

Tofu and Beans Stir-fry

Servings: 2
Preparation Time: 15 minutes

Ingredients:
2 tofu blocks, cut into strips
2 cups garbanzo beans (chick peas)
1 onion, chopped
1 cup carrots, shredded
1 cup green beans, trimmed and chopped
3 tablespoons vegetable oil
¼ cup gluten-free soya sauce
1 tablespoon fresh ginger, grated

2 garlic cloves, minced
3 tablespoons brown sugar
1 tablespoon gluten-free sesame oil
Steamed rice for serving
Vegetable oil for frying

Directions:
1. Heat oil in a wok on medium-high heat. Sauté the onions, ginger, garlic, carrots and green beans until fork tender, about 5-6 minutes. Remove the vegetables from the wok and set aside.
2. Add some more oil to the wok and add the chopped tofu. Fry until golden.
3. Add the garbanzo beans and cooked vegetables to the wok.
4. In a small bowl, mix the soya sauce, sesame oil, and brown sugar. Pour the sauce into the wok and stir to coat well.
5. Serve over steamed rice.

Creamy Chicken

Servings: 4
Preparation Time: 45 minutes

Ingredients:
2 tablespoons vegetable oil

2 cups milk
4 chicken breasts
2 onions, chopped
2 cups tomatoes, diced
2 cups spinach, chopped
2 tablespoons white wine
2 cups chicken broth
¼ cup cheddar cheese

Directions:

1. Pre-heat the oven to 375°FGrill the chicken breasts for 30-35 minutes, until .chicken is cooked through and juices run clear when poked with a fork.
2. Whisk the milk, chicken broth and white wine together in a mixing bowl.
3. Heat oil over medium heat in a large saucepan. Sauté the onions for 1-2 minutes until tender and fragrant.
4. Add tomatoes and spinach and continue sauté for 2-3 more minutes. Add the whisked milk mixture to the sautéed mix and bring to a boil. Reduce heat to medium and let simmer for 10 minutes, uncovered.
5. Pour this preparation over the grilled chicken breasts. Top with cheddar cheese.
6. Place chicken under the broiler until the cheese has melted and is bubbly. Serve immediately.

Beef Broccoli and Pasta

Servings: 4
Preparation Time: 30 minutes

Ingredients:

1 pound lean ground beef

2 tablespoons vegetable oil

2 teaspoons black pepper

1 package of gluten-free noodles like penne or bow ties

2 cups broccoli florets, cooked

1 onion, chopped

2 teaspoons chili powder

1 tablespoon fresh thyme, chopped

2 tablespoons mustard

3 tablespoons mayonnaise

2 tablespoons balsamic vinegar

1-2 tablespoons fresh parsley, chopped

Directions:

1. Heat oil in a pan and brown the ground beef over medium high heat. Remove from heat and drain excess liquids. Add pepper, onion, chili powder, and thyme and continue frying for 3-5 more minutes.
2. Prepare the gluten-free noodles according to package instructions. Place cooked noodle into a serving bowl. Add ground beef and broccoli.
3. In a small bowl, whisk mustard, mayonnaise, vinegar, and parsley together and drizzle it over the noodle mixture. Mix well and serve

Teriyaki Noodles

Servings: 3
Preparation Time: 20 minutes

Ingredients:
¾ cup gluten-free soya sauce
3 tablespoons lemon juice
3 cups rice noodles, cooked
1 cup broccoli, steamed
1 cup cauliflower, steamed
2 cups prawns, steamed
2 teaspoons chili powder

Directions:
1. Boil the soya sauce, lemon and chili powder.
2. Mix the rice noodles, broccoli, cauliflower, and prawns together lightly.
3. Pour the soya sauce mix over the other ingredients and toss together.
4. Serve with a dash of chili powder.

Cheesy Risotto

Servings: 3
Preparation Time: 45 minutes

Ingredients:
2 ¾ cups rice (white or brown), steamed
½ cup tomatoes, chopped
¼ cup onions, chopped
¼ cup garlic, chopped
2 tablespoons dried oregano
Parsley, chopped
¾ cup cheddar cheese, grated
Salt and pepper
¼ cup mixed nuts, finely chopped

Directions:
1. Heat oil in a pan and sauté the steamed rice, tomatoes, onions, garlic, oregano, and parsley.
2. Transfer to a microwavable plate and sprinkle grated cheddar cheese on top. Season with salt and pepper.
3. Heat the mix in a microwave for 15-20 minutes, until cheese is melted.
4. Sprinkle the mixed nuts on top and serve.

Squash and Chili Prawn Dish

Servings: 2
Preparation Time: 20 minutes

Ingredients:

2 tablespoons vegetable oil
10 small prawns, steamed
2 cups squash, cubed
3 teaspoons chili powder
½ cup green bell pepper, chopped
½ cup red bell pepper, chopped
1 small onion, chopped
2 cloves garlic, minced
¼ cup lemon juice
Salt   and   pepper

Directions:
1. Heat oil in a pan and sauté the squash, chili powder, green bell pepper, red bell pepper, onion, garlic and lemon juice for 5 minutes. Add the prawns to heat through.
2. Remove to a serving bowl and season with salt and pepper.

Mustard-Toasted Vegetables

Servings: 4
Preparation Time: 20 minutes

Ingredients:
2 tablespoons olive oil
1 cup potatoes, chopped

1 cup carrots, chopped
2 cups broccoli, chopped
1 cup squash, cubed
2 garlic cloves, minced
¼ cup onions, chopped
½ cup mustard
2 tablespoons honey
Parsley, chopped
½ cup lemon squeeze
Salt and pepper

Directions:
1. Heat oil in a pan and sauté potatoes, carrots, broccoli, squash, garlic, and onions.
2. In a small mixing bowl, mix together the mustard, honey, parsley and lemon juice. Pour over the vegetables and toss to combine.
3. Season with salt and pepper to taste.

Classic Gluten-Free Nachos

Servings: 4
Preparation Time: 15 minutes

Ingredients:
8 cups of gluten-free nachos
2 tablespoons oil
1 cup ground beef

1 cup cheddar cheese, grated
½ cup sour cream
¾ cup tomatoes, chopped
2 teaspoons chili pepper
¼ cup red bell pepper, diced
¼ cup corn kernels

Directions:

1. Heat some oil in a pan and sauté the ground beef until browned. Drain the fat and add the tomatoes, chili pepper, red bell pepper, and corn.
2. Spoon over the nachos and top with grated cheese, Place under the broiler until the cheese is melted.
3. Serve with the sour cream.

DESSERT RECIPES

No-Bake Marshmallow Pudding

Servings: 2
Preparation Time: 10 minutes

Ingredients:
2 bananas, mashed
1 cup chocolate milk
½ cup milk (full cream or low fat)
2 cups mini marshmallows
12 Rice crackers

Directions:
1. Crush the rice crackers.
2. Stir together the mashed bananas, chocolate milk, milk, and marshmallows.
3. Combine mixture with crushed rice crackers then put in shot glasses for serving.

No-Cook Butter Fudge Cookie

Servings: 5
Preparation Time: 20 minutes

Ingredients:
2 cups cookie butter*

2 cups chocolate chips
1 cup condensed milk
½ cup white sugar
2 tablespoons butter, melted
1 teaspoon vanilla extract
½ teaspoon salt

*Cookie butter is a Trader Joe's product. It resembles peanut butter, but tastes like cinnamon cookie dough.

Directions:
1. Heat the condensed milk, sugar and melted butter in a saucepan. Add the chocolate chips, and stir until melted. Bring to a boil and let it simmer for 2-3 minutes.
2. Add this mixture to the cookie butter. Combine thoroughly and add vanilla extract and salt.
3. Refrigerate until set, and serve.

Peanut Butter Squares

Servings: 10 squares
Preparation Time: 80 minutes

Ingredients:
1 cup chocolate chips, melted
2 teaspoons butter, melted

1 cup chunky peanut butter
1 tablespoon sugar (brown or white)
Cinnamon

Directions:
1. Mix melted chocolate chips, butter, peanut butter, and sugar in a saucepan over medium-low heat.
2. Refrigerate for 1 hour, cut into squares, sprinkle with cinnamon, and then serve.

Molasses Cookies

Servings: 15 cookies
Preparation Time: 20 minutes

Ingredients:
3 cups gluten-free flour
2 teaspoons baking soda
1 teaspoon cardamom, ground
1 teaspoon cinnamon, ground
½ cup butter, melted
1 cup molasses
2 eggs

Directions:

1. Mix gluten-free flour, baking soda, cardamom, cinnamon, melted butter, molasses and eggs thoroughly.
2. Preheat the oven to 350°F.
3. Shape the mix in to flattened balls about 1 inch in size, and place them evenly spaced 2" apart on a cookie sheet.
4. Bake for 9-12 minutes, until the edges are golden brown and cookie are cooked through.

Cornflake Mallow Cookie Bars

Servings: 12 cookies
Preparation Time: 30 minutes

Ingredients:
2 cups rice flour
1 teaspoon baking powder
½ teaspoon salt
1 cup butter, melted
½ cup honey or maple syrup
1 egg
2 tablespoons cookie butter
3 cups gluten-free corn flake cereal
2 cups small marshmallows

Directions:

1. Grease a 9 x 13" baking pan, and preheat the oven to 350ºF.
2. Combine the rice flour, baking powder, salt, butter, liquid sweetener, egg, cookie butter, and cornflakes.
3. Spread the mixture in the oven pan, and bake for 15-20 minutes. Cut into squares before serving.

www.ingramcontent.com/pod-product-compliance
Lightning Source LLC
Chambersburg PA
CBHW062133020426
42335CB00013B/1204